Build Strength, Boost Flexib
and Increase Balance
in Just 10 Minutes a Day

28 DAYS
OF
CHAIR YOGA

FOR SENIORS

Ottie Oz

Table of Contents

A Gift to Our Readers

I'm thrilled to include a special gift for our readers
15 Guided Meditations.

These 15 guided voice meditations provide a unique opportunity to enhance your practice. They're designed to be accessible and convenient for your busy lifestyle.

Unlock the power and experience the countless benefits they offer.

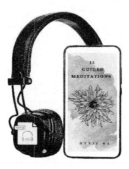

Elevate your practice, enhance your well-being, and embrace the serenity that awaits you.

Scan QR code or go on

chairyoga.littlegeckopublishing.com

Introduction

"Yoga is not about touching your toes.
It is what you learn on the way down."

– Jigar Gor

This transformative guide is created to strengthen your body, increase your mobility, and improve your overall well-being. In 28 days, these routines will empower you to become stronger, leaner, and more balanced—all in less than 10 minutes daily. You will find 28 daily chair yoga routines designed to work on different body parts to help you become stronger and increase your mobility.

Whether you're new to yoga or have been practicing for years, this book is designed with the more mature population in mind. So grab a chair and get ready to discover the incredible benefits of *Chair Yoga for Seniors!*

Staying active becomes even more crucial as we age. Our bodies naturally start to lose muscle mass and bone density. Regular exercise helps maintain strength in our muscles and bones, reducing the risk of falls and fractures. Maintaining our physical fitness and overall health becomes increasingly important. But that doesn't mean we have to surrender to the challenges of time. Instead, we can adapt and discover new ways to nurture our bodies and minds. Chair yoga is one such pathway—a gentle, accessible, and incredibly effective practice tailor-made for people with reduced mobility due to different health conditions. No matter your age, various health conditions can affect you earlier in life, and not all, even young people, can exercise lying on the floor.

Regarding staying active and healthy, chair yoga or any other chair exercises are a game-changer. This gentle exercise offers numerous benefits that can enhance your overall well-being. Chair yoga helps improve flexibility and range of motion. The gentle stretches in seated positions target key muscle groups, helping increase joint mobility and relieve stiffness.

Not only does chair yoga boost physical health, but it also promotes mental wellness. Regular chair yoga sessions help reduce stress levels and improve relaxation. Focusing on deep breathing techniques aids in calming the mind, promoting mindfulness, and reducing anxiety.

Chair yoga is an inclusive practice accommodating individuals with various physical abilities or limitations. Incorporating chair yoga into your routine can enhance balance and stability—a crucial aspect for seniors—reducing the chances of falls or accidents.

It also provides numerous physical, mental, and emotional benefits, such as improved balance, flexibility, and muscle strength, and reduces stressful health by increasing blood circulation and lowering blood pressure.

Engaging in regular physical activity is not only beneficial for the body but also for mental health. In addition to improving memory and concentration, endorphins that boost mood and reduce stress are released when exercising.

Chair yoga provides a gentle yet effective way for anyone to incorporate movement into their daily routine. This form of yoga adapts traditional poses to be performed while seated or using a chair for support.

How Will You Benefit from This Book?

With this book as your guide, you can expect clear instructions accompanied by illustrations for each exercise. In this *28 Days of Chair Yoga*, you will experience many benefits that can significantly enhance your overall well-being. Incorporating movements and stretches into your daily routine will improve your physical health and nurture your mental and emotional wellness. Don't underestimate the power of this modified practice—it can work wonders for your body and mind!

With each day's practice, you'll notice increased flexibility in your muscles and joints. It may also help reduce joint, head, and back pains. The gentle stretching exercise routines in the book will help to alleviate stiffness and promote a better range of motion. This can be especially beneficial for those with limited mobility or who struggle with arthritis or other conditions.

Chair yoga is also an excellent way to improve balance and stability. Maintaining our equilibrium becomes increasingly important as we age to prevent falls and injuries. The various poses in this book target specific muscle groups that support balance, helping to strengthen them over time.

Furthermore, regular chair yoga sessions promote better circulation throughout the body. Moving the body gently while seated improves blood flow, providing essential nutrients to all organs and tissues. This enhanced circulation can lead to improved energy levels and reduced fatigue.

But it's not just physical benefits that make chair yoga so valuable; it also significantly impacts mental well-being. Practicing mindfulness through focused breathing exercises helps calm the mind and reduce stress. It provides an opportunity for relaxation amidst the hustle of everyday life.

With its easy-to-follow routines specifically designed for older adults, it offers immense value both physically and emotionally.

Age should never hinder us from living our best lives! Embrace the benefits of chair yoga and experience a renewed sense of vitality, strength, and inner peace.

Exercise also boosts mental health by reducing symptoms of anxiety and depression while promoting cognitive function. Staying active keeps our minds sharp and improves memory recall.

Another reason why exercise is vital for seniors is its ability to increase mobility and independence. Strong muscles support joint function, making everyday tasks easier to perform without assistance.

Furthermore, regular exercise promotes better sleep patterns, which is crucial for overall health maintenance.

Chair Yoga Misconceptions

Many misconceptions about chair yoga are circulating, and a few of them are present here.

It's Too Easy: One of the common misconceptions is that chair yoga may not provide a challenging workout compared to other forms of exercise. However, this couldn't be further from the truth! Chair Yoga can help build core strength, enhance muscle tone, and boost overall stamina by engaging in controlled movements and focusing on proper breathing techniques. Some people mistakenly believe that chair yoga is not challenging enough to provide real health benefits. While gentle and accessible, chair yoga can be adapted to different fitness levels, and its effectiveness should not be underestimated. The practice can be demanding, depending on the poses and exercises' intensity.

Another incredible aspect of chair yoga is its ability to promote relaxation and reduce stress. Through guided meditation and mindful breathing exercises incorporated into the practice, participants experience improved mental clarity, reduced anxiety, and enhanced emotional well-being.

It's Only for Seniors: While chair yoga is excellent for seniors due to its accessibility and focus on gentle movements, it's not exclusive to this demographic. Chair yoga can benefit people of all ages and fitness levels. Athletes, office workers, and those recovering from injuries or surgery can find value in chair yoga's adaptability.

It's Not a "Real" Form of Yoga: Some believe chair yoga is not authentic because it adapts traditional yoga poses for seated practice. However, chair yoga incorporates the fundamental principles of yoga, including mindfulness, breathing techniques, and the mind-body connection. It's a legitimate and effective form of yoga.

Boring: In reality, chair yoga can be enjoyable and mentally stimulating. It offers opportunities for self-reflection, relaxation, and the development of mindfulness skills. Many practitioners find it a rewarding and calming practice.

And these are just some of them. So, if you're wondering whether chair yoga works, try it yourself! You'll soon discover how this accessible exercise can transform physical health while promoting inner peace and harmony. Give it a chance; remember that to see the improvement, you need time.

So stick to the program and let me know what you think.

Moreover, regular practice of chair yoga has been shown to boost mental well-being by reducing stress levels. It provides an opportunity for relaxation through deep breathing techniques.

How to Use This Book

"Yoga reminds me that everything is connected,
so we must live, act, and breathe with awareness."
— Adrien Mishler

Regardless of whether you decide to follow this program or not and which page you will start from, it's recommended to read this chapter and what you need to start your journey.

28 Days Chair Yoga Program is great for:

- Beginners who want to start practicing chair yoga
- People with reduced mobility
- People who are looking for low-impact exercise but still want to have a workout
- Individuals who are recovering from surgeries or injuries
- Sedentary individuals who want to offset the negative effects of prolonged sitting
- Yoga teachers looking for new ideas and ways to improve routines for their students

If this is something you think is for you, then keep exploring.

This book has 28 sequences and three bonus ones.

Each day, you will perform different sequences. They all have descriptions of what the routine is focused on. The benefit of it is that you can choose which one you prefer to do or simply follow the program.

If a certain day's routine looks challenging or you feel like your joints need attention on that day, then you can switch the days you're working on.

Also, if you feel that you want a longer session, you can always do an extra day or add one of the bonus sequences. Also, you can repeat the same routine twice.

Find what feels good and make this journey your own.

Never push or continue doing poses if you feel pain. This is your body, and only you know what feels right for it. Stop and listen. It's a journey of respect, discovering your potential, and accepting your limits. Some days, we're strong, and some days, we need to be quiet. Do what feels good. Listen to your body and heart. Be who you are when no one is watching.

All 28 routines have pictures at the back of the book. Once you become comfortable and know how to perform the poses, you can use only pictures as your guide.

Each routine includes light warm-up moves. Before you start the routine, sit in the mountain pose position and gather your thoughts—concentrate on your breath and coordinate your breath with the movement. Finish the routine as well in a mountain pose, savoring the fruit of your practice. When you practice, once you're sitting in a mountain pose position, remember a few things to observe when practicing:

Don't lift your shoulders to your ears unless you're doing shoulder shrugs.

Think that you have a lot of space between your earlobes and shoulders; your neck is nice and tall. Your head is aligned above your heart. You sit relaxed yet with your core engaged and your spine straight. Try to do your body's best. Always think about your breath—don't hold it. It must flow at your pace, in and out.

Considerations

Please read before you proceed with the chair yoga routines.

If you are concerned about injuring yourself by practicing chair yoga, the best action is to talk to your doctor or physical therapist. Show them the chair yoga routines you plan to practice and ask them to recommend postures suitable for your health condition.

It's important to remember that yogic postures are eased into slowly, and there is a heightened focus on the body. Try one of the variations if you struggle to ease into an asana. If none of the variations work, skip that asana and move on to the next. You should never be in pain while practicing. If you feel or experience any pain, do not push yourself further.

Another important aspect of being comfortable while in asanas is remembering to breathe. It would be best if you were not holding your breath while in an asana unless directed to do so—and even when required to do so, it should never be longer than a couple of seconds. This is why it would be beneficial to practice breathing exercises every day.

Important things to remember while practicing chair yoga (or yoga of any kind):

- Consistency is the key to achieving your goals. Practice regularly. You will not acquire any results by practicing once every other week.
- You don't have to have the perfect form. Follow the directions to the best of your ability and only to a point where you are comfortable.
- Yoga is not a competition or a race. Work at your own pace and use the best variations for you.
- Pay attention to your head and neck alignment to avoid pain.
- Sit toward the front edge of the chair with your feet flat on the floor, hip-width apart. This position provides stability and allows for better alignment during poses.
- Work on coordinating breath and movement. Listen to your body. You can keep your knees together or apart. Keep arms on your thighs with palms

up or down. There is no right or wrong; there is you and what feels good to you.

- Sit up straight with your spine aligned and shoulders relaxed. Proper posture is essential for safe and effective chair yoga.

- Incorporate mindful breathing throughout your practice. Deep, rhythmic breathing can help you relax and enhance your focus on each pose.

- Drink water before and after your practice to stay hydrated, especially if your session is more prolonged or intense.

- There are recommendations for how many breaths to hold the pose. However, if you want to reduce or add more breaths to your poses—feel free to do so. Don't feel bad if you cannot hold a pose for three breaths. It's not a competition. This is your journey. Holding the position for three breaths might be a challenge initially, but with 20 days of practice, you could comfortably sustain the pose for four breaths. Your body will naturally adapt, desiring to linger in the position for an extended duration.

- Those with **spinal disc problems** or **glaucoma** should take special care to choose postures without twists or inversions. NEVER force yourself into a twisted position, or any position for that matter, using your hands and forcing yourself. When performing forward bending, move from the hip joint without rounding your back. Avoid bouncing and impact.

- Chair yoga is not just about physical movement; it is also about mindfulness and relaxation. Stay present and focus on your breath and sensations throughout the practice.

- Don't let your ego get in the way—listen to your BODY.

- It is better not to have a big meal before practicing chair yoga.

We all have different bodies, and their abilities are different. Some days you will feel better, some days not, and it's OK. There is that hype that every day should be perfect; if it's not, then it's a failure. And then we're getting upset and disappointed with ourselves that we failed. We have failed to have a good day! This is just wild! We must accept that we have bad, mediocre, sound, and perfect days. And when it's a 'bad' day, we take it, move on, and do our best to be the best versions of ourselves. We cannot always be happy, content, and on top of the world, constantly feeling the winners. We don't always feel great physically; we ache and hurt. It's not about having a perfect day; it's about accepting the things that we cannot change and moving on. It's about having the wisdom to identify what we can change and the strength to change it.

If you haven't exercised in years, you cannot expect your body to perform at top-notch ability. However, you can expect your body to get there. Chair yoga is not a competition, and it's not about twisting yourself into a pretzel.

It's about your journey. It's about what you will discover.

Getting Ready for Chair Yoga

An Attitude

Sometimes, people, including myself, lose their motivation or their 'why.' Think of your own; why have you decided to do this program? Once you have your why, then remember it when you feel down or are unwilling to do a routine. Remember that the most challenging thing is to show up for your practice. Once you're on the chair—the hard part is done.

Consistency is key. Regular chair yoga practice can improve your balance and flexibility over time. Aim for short, frequent sessions rather than occasional long ones.

Clothing

You don't need fancy yoga clothing. Don't use this as an excuse not to start the program. You should wear something comfortable that will allow you to move around easily. Sometimes, I do my short morning routines in my pajamas because no one is watching, and I feel like it!

Yoga Mat

You don't necessarily need a yoga mat. However, often, people put a yoga mat under the chair to prevent it from sliding. Also, if you prefer to exercise bare feet, it helps prevent friction.

Chair

You need a sturdy chair with no arms. The absence of arms allows for greater flexibility in movement, and the key is to select a chair that remains steadfast throughout your yoga routine, providing stability without shifting or moving. Choose any regular sturdy chair for exercises; steer clear of folding chairs or those with wheels.

Socks or No Socks?

It's your preference. You can exercise bare feet. If you choose to wear socks, make sure they have a grip on their soles.

Room

You can exercise in any room or use an outside space.

If this is an option, I prefer to open the windows to feel the fresh air getting in. But this is only my preference. This is your practice, your choice.

Ensure you have enough free space around you—no sharp objects, corners, or furniture nearby. The room doesn't have to be furniture-free. However, a tidy space can help create a calming atmosphere for your practice.

Now, let's transition into the practical part of this program. These chair yoga routines enhance your flexibility, balance, and overall well-being. As you go through these exercises, remember to honor your body's limitations and make sure to progress at a comfortable pace. Let's get started to kickstart your chair yoga practice!

Day 1

NECK, SHOULDER, ARMS, AND UPPER BACK RELIEF

This chair yoga routine provides targeted relief for your neck, shoulders, arms, and upper back. Throughout the sequence, you'll engage in gentle movements that focus on loosening tension in these key muscle groups. By incorporating stretches and poses specifically tailored for the upper body, you'll experience improved flexibility and circulation, promoting relaxation, reducing discomfort, and building strength.

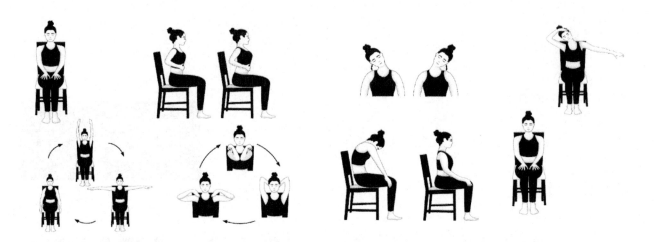

Mountain Pose

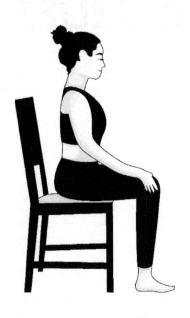

Find a comfortable seated position in the center of the chair, leaving some space between the back of the chair and your back. Rock back and forth until you locate your sit bones. Keep your feet hip-distance apart and flat on the floor. If you prefer, bring your knees together. Take a few deep breaths to center yourself and bring your awareness to the present moment. Begin by gently closing your eyes or softening your gaze. Let go of any distractions and allow your mind to settle. Bring your attention to your breath. Feel the rise and fall of your abdomen with each inhale and exhale. Notice how it feels as it flows in and out of your nose. Follow the breath with your attention, noticing the coolness of the inhale and the warmth of the exhale. Stay for ten breaths, and when ready, move on to the next exercise.

Seated Pelvic Tilt Tuck

Place feet firmly on the floor in mountain pose, arms resting on your knees, and spine erect. Place your hands on top of the pelvis crest to feel the movement. This is a slight movement, just tilting the tailbone back and forth.

Inhale as you tilt the pelvis forward. Exhale as you tilt the pelvis backward. Repeat for six to eight cycles.

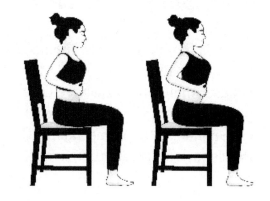

Chair Neck Rolls

Take a couple of deep breaths. Inhale, move your ear toward the right shoulder, and exhale. Make sure that the neck is long, and the shoulders are relaxed and away from the ears. On the inhale, come back to the center, exhale, and pause before switching sides. Repeat on another side, three to five times on both sides.

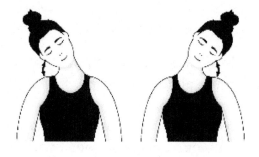

Chair Neck Stretch

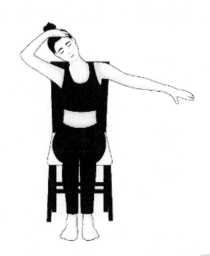

Sit comfortably in the chair, knees stacked over ankles at 90 degrees. Exhale, tilting head right, right hand on left ear, and left arm extended. Inhale, return to center. Exhale, tilt head left, left hand on right ear, and right arm extended. Repeat two more times on both sides.

Chair Mountain Pose Sweeping Arms Flow

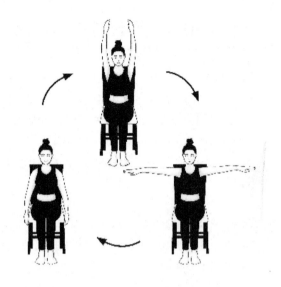

Sit in a mountain pose. Inhale, reaching the arms up, palms facing each other above your head. Exhale and slowly release them down, palms facing down. Inhale, reaching the arms up; exhale with palms facing down. Repeat the sequence for another five times.

Shoulder Socket Rotation

Sit up tall with your back straight. Bring the fingertips to rest on the shoulders.

On the inhale, begin to move the bent elbows from the center, moving upward.

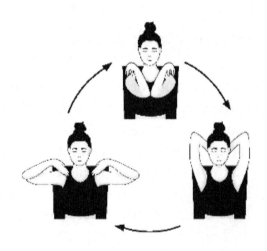

Move them in a circular movement from the center about six times. Repeat the opposite direction another six times. Watch your breath, and work on coordinating the action with your breath at your own pace.

Chair Cat-Cow Pose

Place your arms on your knees. As you inhale, expand your chest, allowing your head and chin to tilt slightly back. On the exhale, round your spine by curling your chest inward. Ensure your shoulders are relaxed and be aware of the space between your shoulders and earlobes. Practice coordinating your breath with the movement, moving at a comfortable pace. Repeat five to eight times.

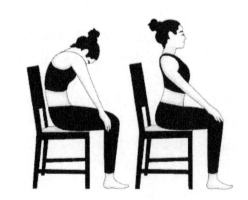

Mountain Pose

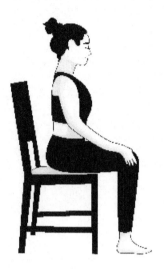

Find a comfortable seated position in the center of the chair, leaving some space between the back of the chair and your back. Take a few deep breaths and say thanks. You've done well.

Day 2

GLUTES, LOWER BACK, AND KNEES STRENGTHENING

Today, you'll engage in a series of movements designed to strengthen and support the glutes, lower back, knees, shoulders, and arms. Focusing on these muscle groups will enhance overall stability and mobility. The routine incorporates poses and stretches that target the glutes and lower back, promoting a stronger core and reduced lower back discomfort.

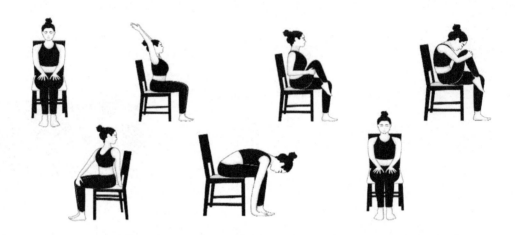

Mountain Pose

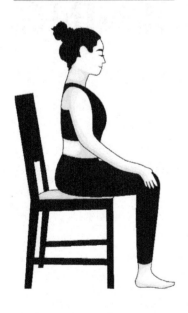

It's your Day 2 when you have shown up for your practice. The hardest part is done. Take a few deep breaths, feel like the air travels into your lungs, and on the exhale, the warm air comes out. Today, you will learn *Right Nostril Breathing Variation Close Up*. This breath practice of the right nostril helps to revitalize the body. It increases the efficiency of the digestive system and also boosts the nervous system, especially the sympathetic nervous system. Close the left nostril with the little finger and ring finger, and breathe in and out through the right. Avoid if blood pressure is high. Do two rounds four times each.

Hands Up Chair

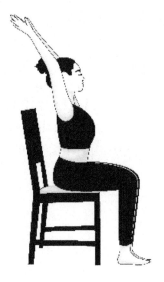

Gently roll your shoulders back, feel your core muscles engaged, and raise your arms above your head on the inhale. Keep shoulders relaxed and away from your ears. Keep the palms facing and touching each other. If not, leave some distance between them; imagine that you're holding a big ball above your head.

If keeping both arms above your head is difficult, bend them slightly through the elbows. Or practice one arm at a time. Keep your arms above your head for a few cycles of breath. Raise your chin slightly, but do not drop your head back. On the exhale, lower your arms. Repeat this cycle two to three times, holding for two to three breaths.

Seated Low Lunge Variation Chair

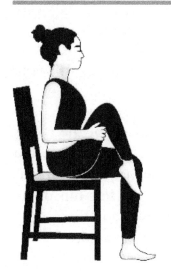

Observe your breath and move from the mountain pose; bend your right knee toward your chest on the inhale. Place your arms behind your thigh and hold the right thigh with your hands while flexing the knee. Try to keep your torso straight, and don't hold your breath.

If you need, lean back for support. Feel the stretch at the hips, lower back, hamstrings, knee, and ankle. Stay in the pose for about three to six breaths. Switch sides.

Knee Head Down Chair

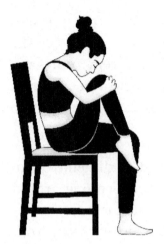

Releasing from the previous pose, inhale, and while you exhale, press the thighs closer to you while you bring the face toward the knee, flexing the neck. Press the thighs, and rest the nose on the knee in the Knee Head Down Chair pose for about three to six breaths. Resting the back completely, make sure you get a grip on the hips and the foot on the floor to avoid slipping from the chair. Repeat the move with the opposite leg.

Chair Seated Twists

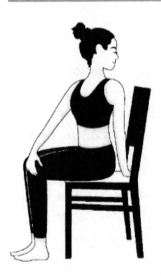

Make sure you're not leaning on the back of the chair. Rock forward and back; find your sit bones. Sit tall with feet touching the floor and knees hip-width apart.

Inhale and place your arms over your head—lift and lengthen.

With the exhalation, twist left from the base of the spine. Your ribcage, shoulders, neck, and eyes go to the left, but the hips remain on the chair. The right hand goes to the left knee, and the left hand is behind the left hip or on the back of the chair. Stay in the position for three deep breaths. Repeat the opposite side, twice each side.

Seated Forward Fold Pose on Chair

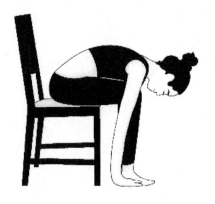

While seated in the mountain pose chair, breathe in deep a few times to relax and extend the spine. Exhaling, bring your arms down toward your feet, with the torso resting on the thighs and chin close to the knees. Stretching the shoulders, place your palms flat on the floor, and remain here for four breaths. As you exhale, push closer into the thighs and abdomen, stretching farther each time. To release, inhale, look up first, then raise your arms before coming back to sit. Remain in the pose for two breaths or till you feel comfortable.

Mountain Pose

Sit for a while, taking deep breaths. Soften your gaze or close your eyes completely. Scan your body for how it feels. Do you feel any tension? Direct your attention to your hands. Begin to move them mindfully, exploring different gestures and motions. Observe the sensations in your fingers, palms, and wrists as you move. Stay present in the experience of this movement. Feel the rise and fall of your abdomen with each inhale and exhale. Complete practice when you feel ready to move on with your daily tasks.

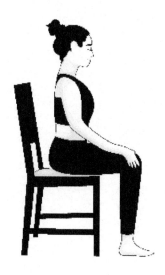

FEET, ANKLES, HAMSTRINGS, AND QUADRICEPS CARE

Dedicate today's chair yoga routine to the well-being of your feet, ankles, hamstrings, and quadriceps. This sequence focuses on providing gentle yet effective stretches and movements to support these crucial muscle groups. You'll improve flexibility, balance, and overall foot health by targeting the feet and ankles. The stretches for hamstrings and quadriceps help maintain proper leg muscle function, allowing for better mobility and reduced tightness.

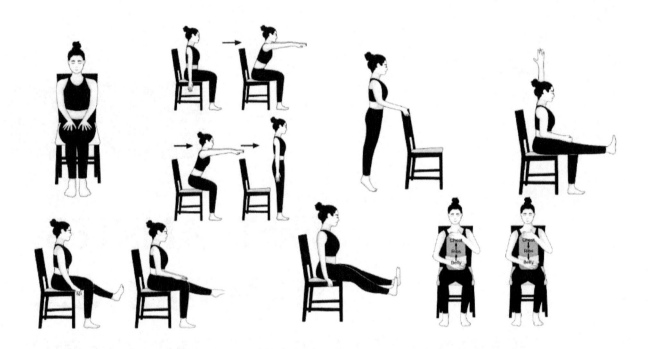

Chair Mountain Pose Stand-Up Flow

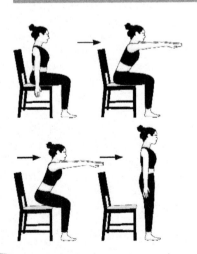

Start in a mountain pose. Feel the rise and fall of your abdomen with each inhale and exhale. Do five rounds, and feel the ground under your feet. Move your toes and feel each of them.

The spine is nice and tall, shoulders rolled back. Reach your arms forward to help you lift your hips off the chair. Hold this position for a couple of breaths; if not, stand up. Feel the ground under your feet. Sit back down with your arms next to you. Repeat five more times.

Heel Raises

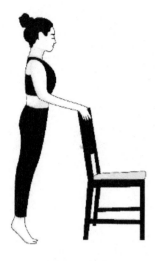

Use the chair's support when attempting heel raises if balance poses a challenge. If this is not an option, then do heel raises when sitting down in a mountain pose.

As you inhale, elevate your body, finding equilibrium on your toes, experiencing the sole's gentle stretch. This sensation extends from the hips, emphasizing a seamless connection to the leg stretch as you gradually rise. Maintain this posture for three to six breaths, then release and repeat. If this is too challenging, you can go up and down, as this is also a great way to stretch your feet.

Easy Pose Chair One Leg Opposite Arm Raised

Sit nice and tall, away from the chair back.

Engage your core, and pull the belly button toward the spine.

Inhale and raise the right leg and left arm. Hold for a few breaths.

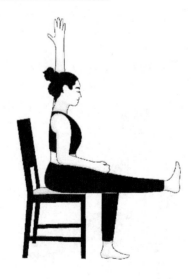

Feel how your leg is activated. Lower the leg or bend through the knee if it's too challenging. Remember to breathe and coordinate movement with breath. Release to the ground after a couple of breaths. Repeat two to three times for each side.

Chair Flexing Foot Pose

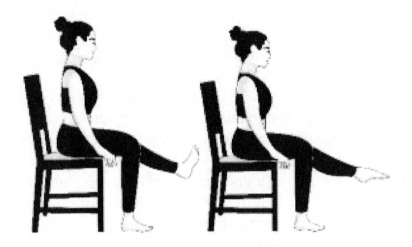

Lift your right leg, and point the toes away from you. As you inhale, lift your toes toward your face and press the heel away. Exhale, and point your toes outward. Repeat this sequence five times before switching to the other leg.

Staff Pose Chair

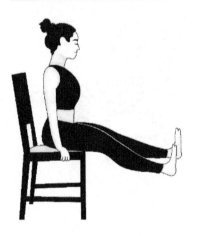

Sit upright with a straight spine and hold onto the sides of the chair seat with both hands. Engage your lower abdomen, and lift both legs simultaneously as you inhale. Keep your legs straight and parallel to the ground, flexing your feet upward. Wiggle your toes to keep your legs active, and if comfortable, hold this position for three breaths. If you cannot lift both legs simultaneously, try to alternate them. As you exhale, gently lower your legs back to the ground and return to a neutral seated position. Repeat it three times, resting in between.

Three-Part Breathing

To end the routine, let's practice a breathing exercise.

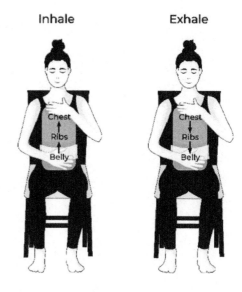

As you begin, you may place your hands on different body parts to feel the air expanding and contracting the area. Begin by inhaling air into your belly, allowing it to expand with each breath in and flatten with each exhale. Take your time to get comfortable with this motion.

Next, take a deep belly breath, and when your belly is expanded, draw in another small breath, and focus it into your lower chest. Place your hand on your lower chest to feel it expand.

When exhaling, first release the air from your chest, then from your belly, allowing both to deflate completely. Practice this until you feel comfortable with the movement.

Now, breathe into your belly, then into your lower chest, and finally, draw in one last breath to fill the upper chest, expanding it up to the collarbone. Feel your entire chest fully expand. When exhaling, start by releasing the air from your upper chest, then from your lower chest, and finally from your belly. Let each part deflate completely before moving on to the next.

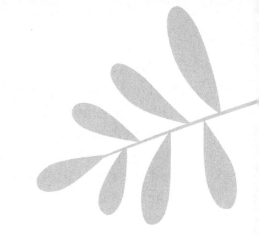

Day 4

SHOULDER AND ARMS MOBILITY

Today's chair yoga routine is dedicated to enhancing shoulder and arm mobility. Through gentle movements and stretches, you'll engage in exercises specifically designed to improve flexibility and strength in these crucial upper body areas. Focusing on the shoulders and arms will promote better posture, alleviate tension, and increase the overall range of motion. Regular practice will contribute to a more comfortable and functional upper body, allowing you to perform daily activities more efficiently. As you dedicate this time to your shoulder and arm well-being, you invest in your overall physical comfort and vitality.

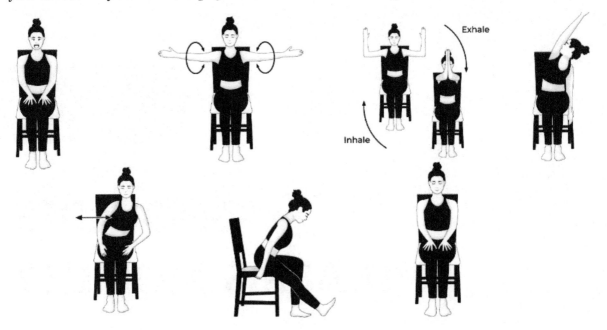

Lion's Breath (Simhasana)

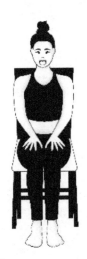

Sit comfortably on the chair and maintain a straight spine. You can lean on your chair backrest—as long as you sit tall with your shoulders lowered.

Unbend your arms and stretch out your fingers. This is to imitate a lion's claws. Inhale through the nostrils, then exhale with a loud "ha" from the mouth, extending your tongue as close to the chin as you can. While breathing out, focus on the middle of your forehead or the end of your nose. Fill up with breath, and go back to neutral facial expression. Repeat four to six times.

Arms to Side Rotations Chair

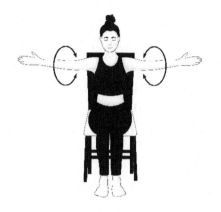

Raise your arms and spread them to the sides parallel to the floor, making a nice T. Breathe in and start making small circles with your wrists in one direction. After a couple of breaths, make a few circles in the opposite direction.

Start making small circles with your arms and slowly increase the motion, making them bigger, and then again, start rotating your arms in the opposite direction, making the circles small until you find stillness.

Seated Cactus Arms Flow Chair

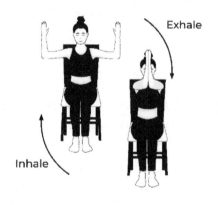

Cactus arms, elbows in line with shoulders, wrists stacked over elbows. Spread the fingers and point them up. Breathe in, and bring your arms to the side with your elbows bent as pictured. Take a deep breath, lift through the chest, and squeeze the shoulder blades together. Listen to your body. As you exhale, bring your elbows, forearms, and hands together. Inhale, open your arms into a cactus position, and squeeze your shoulder blades together. Repeat the flow three to five times. Work on coordinating the flow with the breath.

Chair Seated Side Stretch Pose

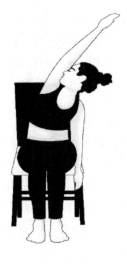

Sit upright. Place the hands on either side of the seat or your lap. Roll your shoulders down the back. Inhale and, pulling in the core, sweep the right arm above the head, creating a lateral bend on the left-hand side. Exhale into the stretch. Allow your chest and head to tilt to the left. Stay in this pose for three breaths. On the inhale, return to the center. Repeat the same with the left side.

You can choose to stay on one side for two to three breaths before switching to the other side, or you may choose to move dynamically between one side and the other on the breath. Do what feels best for your body.

Chair Torso Circles

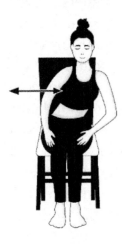

Feel your sit bones firmly grounded to the chair. Inhale, rolling your ribs forward.

Exhale and round your back, ensuring only the torso moves while your legs stay grounded. Draw circles, adjust the size as needed, and listen to your body.

Repeat this movement three to five times at your own breath pace. Change direction and repeat the process.

Half Seated Forward Bend Pose Chair

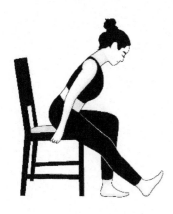

While seated on the chair, move your thighs forward and extend your right leg, placing the foot out and resting it on the heels. Point your toes upward and press the heels firmly to stretch the sole of your foot. Take a moment to feel the sensation of the stretch in the inner sole, and remain in this position, breathing deeply for about three to six breaths. Focus on extending the quads, hamstrings, and calves, feeling release and relaxation in those areas.

Now, repeat the same sequence with the other leg. Pay attention to the leg with more issues and try to hold that stretch a bit longer. You can repeat this stretching process multiple times to work on the tendons and tissues around the plantar fascia (ligament). After completing both legs, take a moment to relax and settle into your seated position.

Day 5

HIP OPENERS, KNEES, UPPER BACK, AND PELVIC RELEASE

Today's practice offers a comprehensive approach to nurturing multiple muscle groups. You'll focus on hip openers, external rotation, knees, shoulders, arms, upper back, and pelvic release. Gentle poses and stretches promote flexibility and relieve tension in these diverse areas. Hip openers and external rotation exercises improve hip mobility, while knee-focused movements support joint health and flexibility. The routine also addresses shoulder, arm, and upper back comfort, reducing muscle tightness and promoting relaxation.

Additionally, pelvic release poses benefit your core and lower back, enhancing overall posture and stability. By engaging in this well-rounded practice, you'll experience improved mobility, reduced discomfort, and enhanced body awareness. Take time to care for these interconnected muscle groups, fostering a sense of balance and harmony throughout your body.

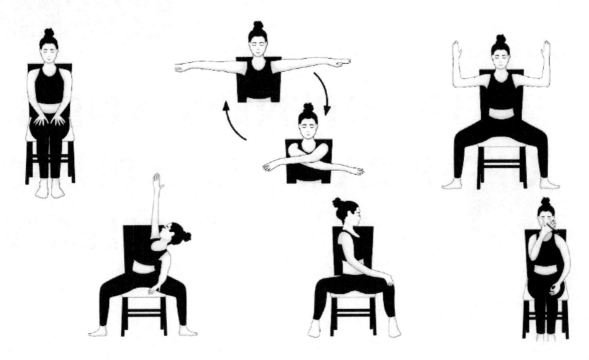

Let's begin in a mountain pose with your arms pressed against your chest.

Take a few deep breaths and become aware of your surroundings. Breathe in, identify the smell, listen carefully, and identify what you can hear around you. Now, shift your focus to your body. Start from your toes, and slowly scan your way up, paying attention to any sensations, tensions, or areas of tightness that you may feel. Take a few moments to breathe into those areas and release any tension or discomfort. When ready—move on to the next step.

Arms Swing Pose Flow Close Up

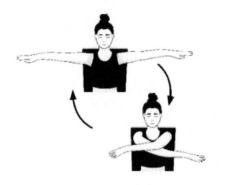

Exercises like arm swings warm up and stretch the shoulders, arms, chest, and upper back, preparing the muscles, tendons, and joints for other poses. Raise your arms sideways, parallel to the floor. Allow your arms to swing forward, hands crossing over each other. Swing arms back, then forward again, alternating which hand swings over the top of the other. This movement may not be in time with your breath, and that is okay. Continue the movement for three to five breaths. You can repeat it twice.

Goddess Pose on Chair

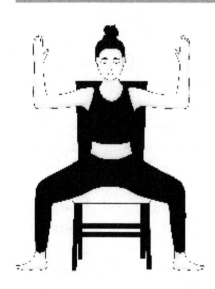

Sit comfortably in the middle of the chair, ensuring there is some space between your back and the backrest. Open your legs wide, keeping your knees aligned over your ankles with your toes slightly turned out. Press through your sit bones and feel grounded through all four corners of your feet. Lengthen your spine and maintain an upright posture. Extend your arms and bend at the elbows, creating a cactus pose with palms facing forward. Slightly squeeze your shoulder blades together. Lift your chest up and outward, feeling the engagement of your shoulder blades and the opening of your heart. To maintain an active stance, gently press through your heels and continue squeezing your shoulder blades. Repeat this sequence for a couple of breath cycles, then lower your arms and repeat the entire process three more times. Keep focusing on your breath and the alignment of your body as you embrace the openness and strength of this pose.

Goddess Pose Chair Side Stretch

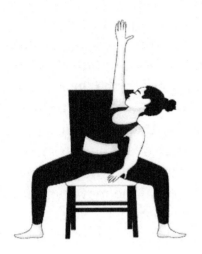

Open your legs wide with feet firmly grounded and pointing outward.

Place your right elbow on your right thigh, palm facing upward. Inhale and sweep your left arm up, gazing at your hand and looking up if possible.

Take three deep breaths in this position. Repeat the same sequence on the other side.

Chair Wide Legged Seated Twist

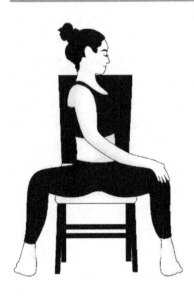

Remain seated in a goddess pose with arms lowered and with your knees wide open. Turn your toes slightly to face them forward and stack your knees over your ankles. Tuck your tailbone in. Both arms are resting on your thighs. Breathe in, lengthening your spine, and twist toward the right.

The twist begins in your belly, ribs, and chest. Your head is last to turn. The left hand goes onto your right knee and your right hand to the back of the chair. Breathe into the twist. Stay here for three deep breaths. Exhale to release and return to the center. Repeat on the opposite side, each side twice.

Alternate Nostril Breathing Chair

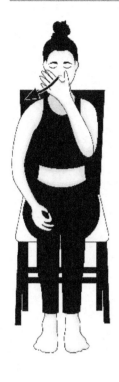

Sit nice and tall in a mountain pose. Rest your left hand on your left thigh or in your lap, or use it to support the elbow of your right arm. Close your right nostril with the thumb of that hand, inhale through the left, and then close it off with your ring finger and pinky. Exhale through the right nostril for a short pause before repeating this cycle three to five times with both nostrils. When finished, return to regular breathing.

When you finish this practice, sit with your eyes closed and your hands in your lap for a few minutes. Let your shoulders fall down and away from your ears. Check how you feel. Breathe in through your nose and exhale through your mouth. Breathe in and feel the air traveling through your throat and to your belly. Open your mouth and exhale.

Feel the sensations in your body right now. Warmth. Coolness. Tingling. Tightness. Pulsation. Relaxation. Hunger. Fullness. Observe the sensations in your body in this moment with patience and kindness. Explore both strong and subtle sensations with curiosity.

Day 6

SHOULDER, ARMS, AND WRIST EXERCISES

With today's well-rounded approach, you'll engage in targeted exercises that enhance the mobility and strength of your shoulders, arms, and wrists. You'll promote flexibility through gentle movements and stretches while building stability in these upper body areas. The routine includes poses to alleviate tension, improve range of motion, reduce muscle tightness, and enhance joint health.

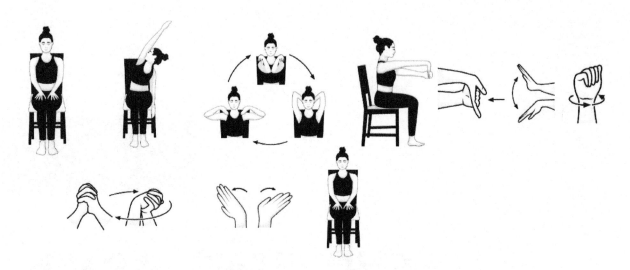

Begin in a mountain pose. You can lean to the back of the chair; however, keep your spine straight, shoulders lowered, and head above your heart. Keep your feet flat on the ground and your spine tall. Softly close your eyes or gaze downward to minimize distractions. Take a deep breath and exhale slowly. Start concentrating on your breath. Notice the sensation. Focus solely on your breath. Scan your body for any tension or discomfort, relaxing those areas with each breath. Engage your hands, moving them mindfully and feeling the sensations in your fingers and palms. Bring your focus back to your breath, following its natural flow in and out of your body. Visualize a warm, radiant light at a chosen point within your body, bringing tranquility to your entire being. Take a few more deep breaths, gradually returning your attention to the present moment. Open your eyes gently, taking a moment to appreciate the calmness and clarity you've cultivated.

Chair Seated Side Stretch Pose

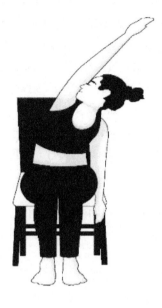

Sit upright. Place the hands on either side of the seat or your lap. Roll your shoulders down the back. Inhale and, pulling in the core, sweep the right arm above the head, creating a lateral bend on the left-hand side. Exhale into the stretch. Allow your chest and head to tilt to the left. Stay in this pose for three breaths.

On the inhale, return to the center. Repeat the same with the left side.

You can choose to stay on one side for two to three breaths before switching to the other side, or you may choose to move dynamically between one side and the other on the breath. Do what feels best for your body.

Shoulder Socket Rotation

Sit up tall with your back straight. Bring the fingertips to rest on the shoulders.

On the inhale, begin to move the bent elbows from the center, moving upward. Move them in a circular movement from the center about six times.

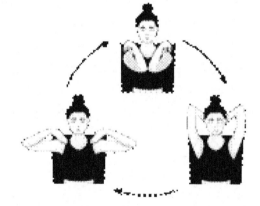

Repeat the opposite direction another six times. Watch your breath, and work on coordinating the action with your breath at your own pace. While practicing, pay attention to your breath and try to coordinate the movement with your breath at your own comfortable pace.

Wrist Flexion Stretch

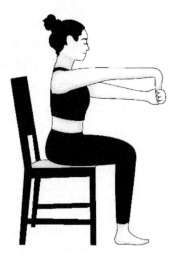

Inhale and extend your right arm straight out, palm facing down. Let your left hand take your right arm's fingers and gently pull them toward your chest. You may feel a stretch on top of your forearm. Stay here for three more breaths, gently going deeper into the stretch on each exhale while respecting your wrist's natural range of movement. Stretch as far as you comfortably can without pain.

Then, pull the fingers to the opposite side—fingers facing up. Repeat the same with your left arm.

Now inhale and extend your right arm straight out, palm facing and opened up. Let 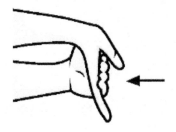 your left hand take your right arm's fingers and gently pull them toward your chest.

Carry on with wrist bending

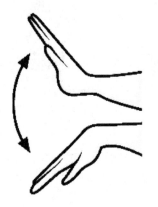

Bring the palms to face in the front with the fingers pointing upward.

Exhale, drop the fingers down as you flex the wrists of both hands. Inhale and raise them palm up, pointing the fingers up, and exhale to drop them down. Repeat this movement about six times, coordinating with the breath. Release and relax, bringing the arms down to the side, standing in mountain pose. Make sure the arms are stretched out and not bent at the elbows, and they are at shoulder level.

Wrist Joint Rotation

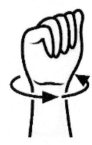

Rotate the right wrist clockwise—about ten times. Rotate the right wrist anticlockwise—about ten times. Repeat the same on the other side. Keep the arms stretched out.

Wrist Rolls Exercise Hands Clasped

Interlace your fingers and rotate your wrists gently at your own pace. Take a few low belly breaths here.

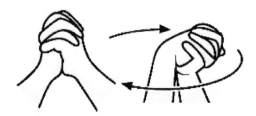

Wrist Exercise Side to Side Close Up

After rotating your wrists, point your fingers up straight, and move your wrist to the left and then to the right. Repeat for both hands. Breathe in and notice if your shoulders remain in the same position or try to move. Only the wrist should be moving. Once the session is completed, close your eyes or soften your gaze. Notice your breath and how your body feels. Take a moment to thank yourself for carving out some time.

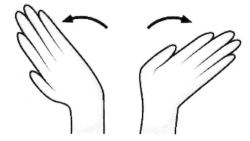

LOWER BACK, HAMSTRINGS, AND NECK RELAXATION

You'll target interconnected muscle groups of the lower back, shoulders, arms, hamstrings, and neck through gentle poses and stretches to release tension and promote a sense of ease. They often accumulate stress from daily activities.

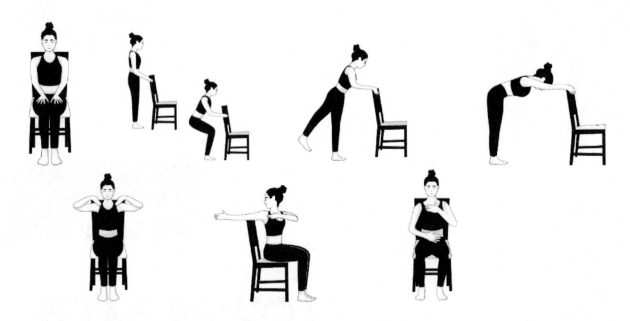

Mountain Pose Chair to Chair Pose Flow

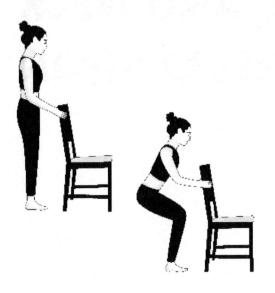

Stand at the back of the chair, holding onto the sides of the chair if help with balance is needed. Take a few deep breaths. Notice how you feel. Feel your ribs, inhale, and slowly exhale. Inhale, stand tall, grounding down into the soles of the feet and extending the spine upward. Exhale, sit weight back into heels. If you need a bigger challenge—your toes can be lifted to exaggerate the weight in the heels. Lower belly pulled in. The knees should be positioned behind the toes. Keep length in the spine and the back of the neck. Hold for three breaths. Repeat three times.

Mountain Pose Chair One Leg Backlit

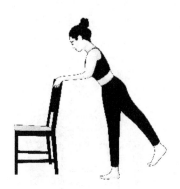

Keep your hands on the back of the chair. Stand tall. Bring your weight to the right foot. Extend the left leg back and lift off the ground. The toes of both feet are pointing forward. Move back and forth for three breaths, or you can hold it for three breaths. Repeat with the opposite leg. Repeat twice on each side.

Standing Forward Bend Chair

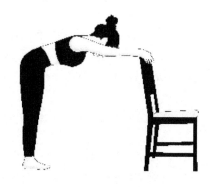

Stand in front of the chair in a standing mountain pose with your legs straight and fully stretched. Pull your kneecaps up. On the inhale, raise your arms toward the ceiling with your palms facing forward. Stretch your whole body. Take one or two breaths. On the exhale, bend forward from the waist. Keep your legs fully stretched. Make sure your body weight is placed equally on both feet. Keep the palms gently pressed, and do not push the body weight on the chair. Keep the length on the back, and fully extend the spine so that it is parallel to the floor. Hold the pose for three to five breaths. Repeat two sets of the practice.

Chair Seated Shoulder Circles

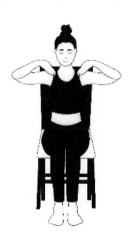

Sit on the chair facing forward, feet hip-distance apart or together on the floor. Inhale, lift your arms to the side, parallel to the floor. Exhale, and bring fingertips to shoulders. Begin to circle in one direction. Circles can be large or small. Pause, and bring attention to your breathing. Circle six to eight times in each direction. Keep your spine straight. Pause, inhale to open arms out, exhale lower arms down, and bring it to the center.

Seated Twist Arms Shoulder Level Pose Chair

Sit up nice and tall. Keep some distance between the chair's backrest and your back. Let the back be straight and long, feet grounded, and ankles and knees in one straight line. Keep the feet together or apart. Extend both arms to the sides in line with the shoulders, palms facing forward.

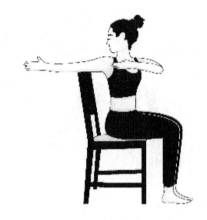

As you inhale, root the sit bones on the chair and lengthen the spine (imagine you are creating space between your vertebrae).

Exhale, twist to the right side originating from the lower back, taking the right hand to the back as far as possible and the left palm on the right shoulder.

Keep your gaze on the right hand by gently and comfortably turning the neck.

Stay here for three to five deep breaths. Keep twisting slightly more with every exhalation (as much as possible without any strain) without moving the lower body.

Mountain Pose

Find a comfortable seated position in the center of the chair, leaving some space between the back of the chair and your back. Rock back and forth until you locate your sit bones. Keep your feet hip-distance apart and flat on the floor. If you prefer, bring your knees together. Close your eyes or soften your gaze. Bring your attention to your breath, feeling the rise and fall of your chest and the expansion and contraction of your abdomen. Inhale deeply in and out. Inhale while counting to four, hold your breath for four, and exhale, counting to six. If these intervals are too long, do three, three, and four. Continue this rhythmic breathing for two minutes, allowing your body and mind to relax.

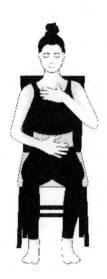

Day 8

HAMSTRINGS, HIP OPENERS, QUADRICEPS, AND UPPER BACK FLOW

Welcome to Day 8 of your chair yoga journey! This routine is designed to flow seamlessly through poses focusing on the hamstrings, heart openers, hip openers, quadriceps, and upper back. This sequence will nurture these vital muscle groups' flexibility, mobility, and balance.

The routine includes heart-opening poses to foster a sense of expansion and vitality, while hip and hamstring stretches promote ease of movement and reduce tightness. Quadriceps engagement and upper back stretch improve muscle functionality and posture.

You'll experience improved circulation, increased flexibility, and a deeper connection to your body through regular practice.

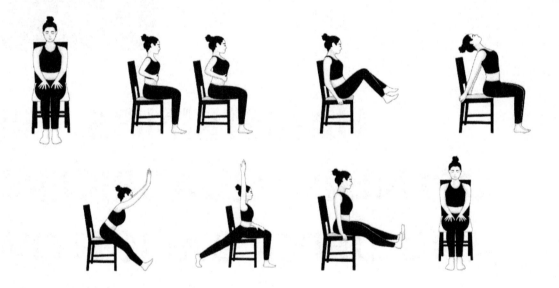

Seated Pelvic Tilt Tuck

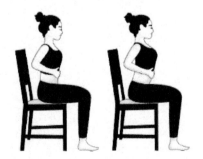

Place feet firmly on the floor in mountain pose, arms resting on your knees, and spine erect. Take a few deep breaths, put your arms on the tummy, and feel it rising and falling. Become aware of your surroundings. What can you hear? What can you smell? How do you feel? Are your shoulders lowered? Are your abdominals engaged? Do you feel the ground under your feet?

Place your hands on top of the pelvis crest to feel the movement. This is a slight movement, just tilting the tailbone back and forth. Inhale as you tilt the pelvis forward, like tipping a bowl full of water ahead. Exhale as you tilt the pelvis backward. Repeat for six to eight cycles.

Boat Pose Variation on Chair

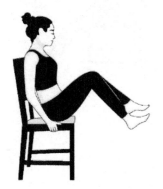

Sit straight and, on the inhale, grab the sides of the chair with your hands, positioning them right behind your buttocks. Curl your four fingers underneath the chair while resting your thumbs near the buttocks. Your weight should be on the outer edges of your palms. As you exhale, lift your feet off the floor while keeping your knees bent. Squeeze your inner thighs to keep your legs together and cross your ankles, aligning them with the chair seat.

Inhale and lengthen your spine as you engage your core and draw your abdomen to bear the weight of your legs. You'll naturally lean back, maintaining an open chest while using your hands on the chair for balance and reducing pressure on the lower back. Stay in this position for two to four breaths, rest, and repeat it again.

Cobra Pose Chair

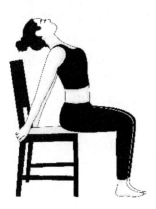

Begin by sitting up tall at the edge of the chair, ensuring your shoulders are relaxed. Open your chest and squeeze your shoulder blades together as you look upward.

Inhale deeply and take your arms behind you, holding onto the chair for support. Lift your chest and shoulders, gazing upward toward the sky with your chin slightly tilted. Remain here for three to six slow and deep breaths. If you like, repeat the sequence for a second round, staying in the pose for another set of breaths.

Seated Downward Facing Dog Pose Chair

Extend the legs—one at a time. On the inhale, flex the feet toward yourself. Extend the arms up, exhale to lean forward slightly from the hips, hugging the navel in. Think of keeping your back flat. Scoot the sit bones back to help balance. Keep the neck long. Bend your knees slightly if needed. Stay in this position for a few breaths. If required, take a break, and repeat it.

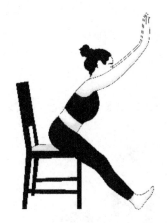

If this pose is not doable, with both legs stretched out, then alternate legs. Pay attention to the leg with more issues and try to hold that stretch a bit longer. After completing both legs, release the stretch and sit back, resting your feet on the floor.

Warrior Pose I Chair Variation

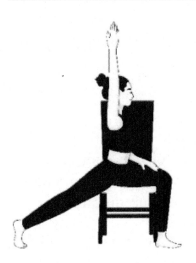

Slide your left leg toward the left side. Let the left leg rest over the edge of the chair while swinging your right leg behind you. Position the sole of your left foot on the floor, roughly parallel to the chair's seat. Straighten your right leg, using your toes for support. If needed, you can slightly bend your right knee. Your upper body is turned toward the left leg, creating a pleasing 90-degree angle with your knee stacked above the ankle. Engage your pelvis, ensuring a straight spine, and lift your heart upward. On an inhale, raise your right arm toward the ceiling while allowing your left forearm to rest on your thigh. Take two to three breaths and repeat on another side.

Staff Pose Chair

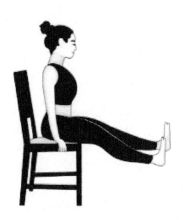

Sit upright with a straight spine and hold onto the sides of the chair seat with both hands. Engage your lower abdomen, and lift both legs simultaneously as you inhale. Keep your legs straight and parallel to the ground, flexing your feet upward. Wiggle your toes to keep your legs active, and if comfortable, hold this position for three breaths. If you cannot lift both legs simultaneously, try to alternate them. As you exhale, gently lower your legs back to the ground and return to a neutral seated position. Repeat it three times, resting in between.

Before you get on with your daily life, sit quietly and absorb the goodness of your practice.

Day 9

EMPOWERING LOWER BACK, NECK, SHOULDERS, ARMS, AND UPPER BACK

Congratulations on reaching Day 9 of your chair yoga journey! Today's routine empowers and rejuvenates your lower back, neck, shoulders, arms, and upper back. With each movement, you're taking a step toward greater well-being and vitality.

As you engage in poses targeting the lower back, you'll strengthen and release tension, promoting a healthier spine. Gentle stretches for the neck, shoulders, arms, and upper back will melt away stress, fostering a sense of ease and relaxation.

Remember, every moment you dedicate to self-care is an investment in your physical and mental health. Embrace the challenge and embrace the rewards that this routine brings. As you move through the poses, visualize the energy flowing through your body, revitalizing each muscle group.

Stay committed, and you'll experience the benefits of increased flexibility, reduced discomfort, and improved posture. Your journey is a testament to your dedication to well-being, and each practice brings you closer to a more vibrant and balanced you. Keep up the great work!

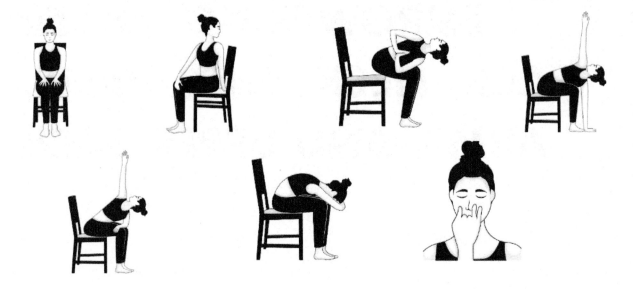

Sit nice and tall. Make sure you're not leaning on the back of the chair. Rock forward and back; find your sit bones. Sit tall with feet touching the floor and knees hip-width apart. Become aware of your breath, and when ready, move on to the next step.

Chair Seated Twists

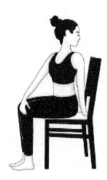

Inhale and place your arms over your head—lift and lengthen. With the exhalation, twist left from the base of the spine. Your ribcage, shoulders, neck, and eyes go to the left, but the hips remain on the chair. The right hand goes to the left knee, and the left hand is behind the left hip or on the back of the chair. Stay in the position for three deep breaths. Repeat the opposite side. Twice each side. Keep your shoulders away from the ears.

Revolved Chair Pose Hovering above Chair

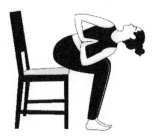

Breathe in as you stand firmly on your feet, gently bending your knees, with palms put together against your chest. Upon exhaling, gently lower your hips while maintaining a slight distance from the chair. Inhale again, and as you do, gracefully twist your chest and shoulders to the right, bringing your palms together in front of your heart.

Find yourself in the revolved chair pose, hovering over the chair for approximately three complete breath cycles. If you find it more comfortable, you can also perform this variation while seated on the chair. Once you've relished the sensation, smoothly transition to the other side, allowing the same sequence to flow in the opposite direction.

Revolved Chair Pose Chair

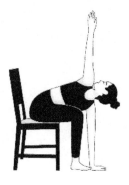

Start in a mountain pose with your spine straight and roll back the shoulders. Inhale and extend the spine, exhale, and bend forward, reaching for the ground with the left arm. Rest your palm on the floor; if this is not possible, lean onto your fingers or rest your left elbow on the top of your knees. The core is active and supports you, too. Inhale as you raise the right arm up and exhale, looking up at the extended limb. Stay here for two to three deep breaths and repeat on another side.

Seated Half Forward Fold Pose Chair

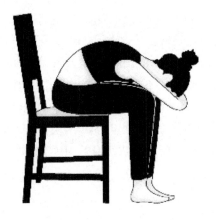

While seated in the mountain pose, breathe in deep for a few times to relax and extend the spine. Exhaling, fold your arms above your knees and allow your head to rest on your forearms. Feel your feet on the floor. Repeat this process as needed for a longer duration. If you need help, use a cushion for extra support under your chest and diaphragm. The aim is to release the tension and open the lower back. Breathe, listen to your body, and choose the position that you feel comfortable in. Stay for three to five breaths.

Alternate Nostril Breathing

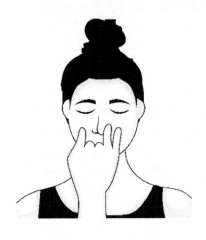

Sit comfortably in a mountain pose. Nadi shodhana, or alternate nostril breathing, is exactly as it sounds: breath control through breathing through alternating nostrils. The technique goes as follows:

Sit in a comfortable position. Each breath will be inhaled and exhaled through the nose. Bring your hand up to your nose, resting your thumb and ring finger on either side of your nose lightly without closing your nostrils. First, press your thumb against your right nostril, closing it. Exhale slowly and fully through your left nostril. Release your right nostril and press your ring finger against your left nostril, closing it. Inhale slowly and deeply. Release your left nostril and press your thumb back down on your right nostril. Repeat this process throughout the breathing exercise.

ABDOMINALS, HIP OPENERS, KNEES, QUADRICEPS, AND UPPER BACK REVITALIZATION

You've reached a milestone—Day 10 of your chair yoga exploration! Today's invigorating routine targets your abdominals, hip openers, knees, quadriceps, and upper back. This practice celebrates your commitment to self-care and your journey toward a healthier you.

Engage in poses that activate your abdominals, fostering core strength and stability. Explore hip openers that enhance flexibility and encourage a free flow of energy. Gentle stretches for knees, quadriceps, and the upper back create a harmonious blend of muscle care and revitalization.

You've come so far; this routine is a testament to your dedication. As you embrace these poses, embrace your journey—one that leads to increased vitality, reduced tension, and a deeper connection to your body. Keep moving forward with confidence and enthusiasm!

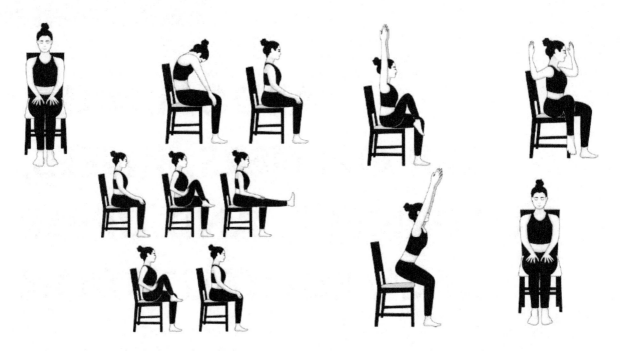

Before moving on to the cat-cow pose, let's practice left nostril breathing. We've already practiced right nostril breathing, so we will do the same—just with the left.

Left Nostril Breathing Variation Close Up: This breath practice of the left nostril enhances circulation to the right hemisphere of the brain, triggering heightened creativity, intuition, and emotional intelligence. Close the right nostril with the little finger and ring finger and breathe in and out through the left. Avoid if blood pressure is high. Do two rounds ten times each.

Chair Cat-Cow Pose

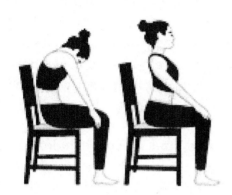

Place your arms on your knees.

As you inhale, expand your chest, allowing your head and chin to tilt slightly back. On the exhale, round your spine by curling your chest inward. Ensure your shoulders are relaxed, and be aware of the space between your shoulders and earlobes.

Practice coordinating your breath with the movement, moving at a comfortable pace. Repeat five to eight times.

Remember to smile, inhale deeply, and repeat this movement three to five times. Take your time and enjoy the practice.

Seated Low Lunge Variation Chair Arms Raised

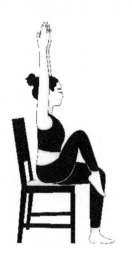

Sit tall with the spine extended. Engage your core. Notice all the muscles that take part in it when you cough. Engage the core with the belly button pulled in. Raise both your arms and lift one leg and exhale to lower the leg. Repeat the opposite side. Repeat six times for each leg.

Seated External Hip Rotation Pose Cactus Arms Chair

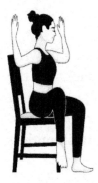

Sit upright, ensuring your shoulders are relaxed and your spine remains straight. Feel a sense of grounding through your hips and feet. Position your arms in a cactus shape, aligning your elbows with your shoulder and stacking your wrists above your elbows. Spread your fingers wide and direct them upward. Inhale, sweep your arms to the sides while keeping your elbows bent, as shown. As you breathe in, engage your core muscles, lengthen your neck, and draw your shoulder blades down your back.

With an inhale, extend your right leg to the right side, and as you exhale, bring it back to the center. Repeat this motion eight to ten times with one leg. If your arms feel fatigued, release the cactus arm position, and take a few breaths in the mountain pose. Then, repeat the sequence on the other side.

Seated Low Lunge Pose

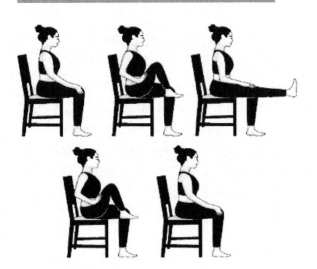

This easy flow will help stretch your feet, ankles, hips, and knees and strengthen your pelvic floor. Sit tall with both feet on the floor and sit bones grounded on the chair. Inhale, and bend your right knee toward your chest.

Exhale, and extend your leg out. Toes up toward the ceiling. Inhale, and bring it back by bending your right knee toward your chest. Exhale, and place your foot on the floor. Repeat on the other side—a total of five times for each leg. If you need to bend your knee toward your chest, you can grab under the knee and support your move.

Chair Pose Hovering Above Chair

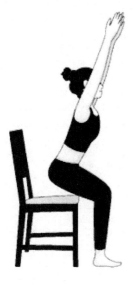

Maintain an upright posture and lift your arms above your head while exhaling deeply. Inhale and move into a chair pose, gently raising yourself to your feet above the chair. Inhale through your nose and exhale audibly through your mouth. Exhale and return to a seated position, arms still extended overhead. Inhale again and resume the chair pose. Repeat this sequence six times.

Come back to the chair mountain pose. Feel the ground under your feet.

Breathe in through your nose. Allow your lungs to fill with air. Feel your chest and abdomen rise as you inhale slowly and steadily. Hold your breath for a moment at the top of your inhale. Exhale through your mouth slowly. Focus on your sensations as you breathe—the rise and fall of your chest and the peaceful rhythm of your inhales and exhales. Let go of any thoughts or distractions, allowing your body and mind to relax. Absorb all the good of your session.

UPPER BACK, HIP, PELVIC, SHOULDER, AND ARM HARMONY

Welcome to Day 11 of your chair yoga series! This routine focuses on creating a harmonious balance in your upper back, hips, pelvic area, shoulders, and arms. You'll nurture these interconnected muscle groups through purposeful poses and stretches for improved well-being.

Experience gentle movements that address tension in the upper back, promoting relaxation and comfort. Hip and pelvic stretches encourage fluidity in movement and increased mobility. The routine includes shoulder and arm engagement, contributing to overall upper-body strength and alignment.

As you engage in this practice, please take a moment to connect with your body and its sensations. With each movement, you're promoting balance and vitality within yourself. Regular participation in these routines adds to your overall wellness journey, helping you create a more harmonious connection between body and mind.

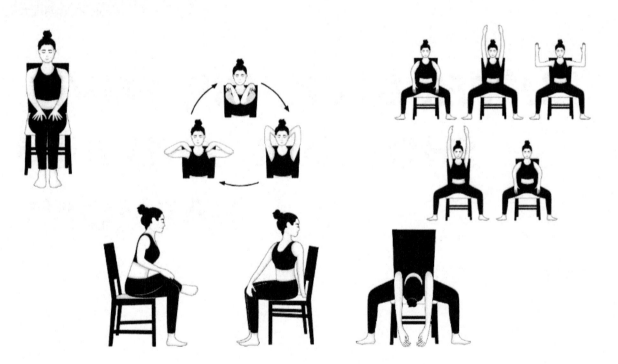

Mountain Pose

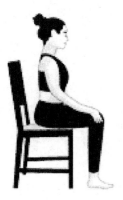

Find a comfortable seated position in the center of the chair, leaving some space between the back of the chair and your back. Rock back and forth until you locate your sit bones. Keep your feet hip-distance apart and flat on the floor. If you prefer, bring your knees together. Close your eyes or soften your gaze. Bring your attention to your breath, feeling the rise and fall of your chest and the expansion and contraction of your abdomen. Inhale deeply in and out. Inhale while counting to four, hold your breath for four, and exhale, counting to six. If these intervals are too long, do three, three, and four. Continue this rhythmic breathing for two minutes, allowing your body and mind to relax.

Shoulder Socket Rotation

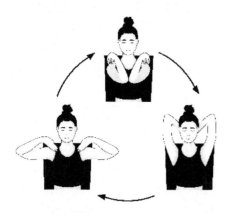

With the elbows bent, shoulder rolls strengthen the rotator cuff muscles, strengthening the shoulder joint. In addition to preventing injuries, this provides a solid foundation for poses requiring shoulder strength. Shoulder rolls with bent elbows can effectively aid in combating diseases and ailments caused by aging, such as osteoporosis and rheumatoid arthritis.

Move them in a circular movement from the center about six times. Repeat the opposite direction.

Goddess Pose on Chair Arms Flow

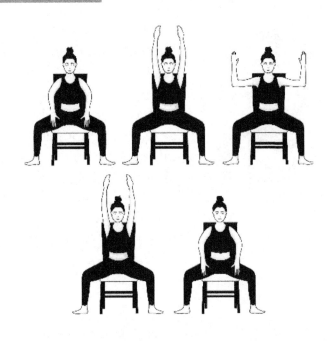

Inhale to rotate the hips outward, bringing the feet to 120 degrees, with toes pointing sideways and knees bent. Gently push out the inner thighs as you plant both feet firmly on the floor. Raise your arms overhead—palms facing each other—keeping shoulders away from ears. Exhale while bending elbows so forearms are perpendicular and palms are facing forward (cactus arms). Hold for three to fove breaths before inhaling to extend arms up again with palms together. Lower arms back down at shoulder level in an exhale, and place hands on inner thighs before inhaling again to raise them. Complete four to six repetitions of this flow, coordinating breathing as needed, then release and relax.

Chair Pigeon Pose

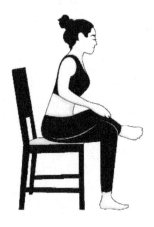

Sit nice and tall, with your back straight. Now, take a deep breath in as you lift your right leg, holding it gently with your hands, and position it over your left thigh, finding a comfortable sitting position. This seated chair pigeon pose serves to enhance the flexibility and fitness of your hip joint and knee through controlled movement. Once settled into the pose, aim to maintain an erect posture, and take three deep breaths or as many as you require to feel at ease. If you encounter difficulty in crossing one leg over the other, alternatively, lift your right leg, cradling it in your arms for a few seconds before gradually releasing it. Repeat this sequence on the opposite side. Repeat it twice on each side.

Chair Seated Twists

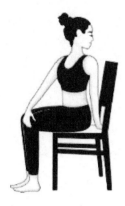

Make sure you're not leaning on the back of the chair. Rock forward and back; find your sit bones. Sit tall with feet touching the floor and knees hip-width apart.

Inhale and place your arms over your head—lift and lengthen. With the exhalation, twist left from the base of the spine. Your ribcage, shoulders, neck, and eyes go to the left, but the hips remain on the chair. The right hand goes to the left knee, and the left hand is behind the left hip or on the back of the chair. Stay in the position for three deep breaths. Repeat the opposite side. Twice each side.

Wide Legged Forward Bend Pose Chair Hands Floor

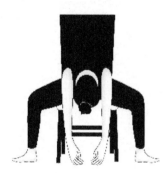

Open legs wide, keeping knees and toes in the same direction. Stack your knees over your ankles. Ground through all four corners of feet. Inhale and raise arms overhead. On the exhale, fold forward. Listen to your body and go as low as your body lets you. It doesn't matter if it's only a few inches. You can use blocks or a stack of books to bring the floor closer to you. Stay here for three deep breaths. If you're comfortable—remain for longer.

Let's complete the session with *Cooling Breath.*

Sit comfortably. Close your eyes gently if you're comfortable doing so, and take a few deep breaths to center yourself. Curl your tongue lengthwise into a "U" shape; if you can't, you can make an "O" shape with your lips. Inhale slowly and deeply through the curled tongue or lips as if you are sipping in cool air. Imagine that you are drawing in a refreshing breeze. After a full inhalation, close your mouth. Exhale slowly and thoroughly through your nose. Continue this cycle, inhaling through the curled tongue or lips and exhaling through the nose for 5 –10 breaths or as long as it feels comfortable. Feel the cooling sensation as you inhale and the calming effect as you exhale. After you've completed the *Cooling Breath* (Sitali Pranayama), return to normal breathing with your mouth closed.

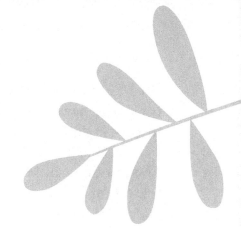

Day 12

PSOAS RELEASE FOR UPPER BACK COMFORT

On Day 12, you'll focus on nurturing your pelvic muscles and relieving your upper back. The psoas muscle is critical in connecting your upper and lower body, aiding in core stability, posture improvement, and overall movement.

This routine will help you to release tension in the shoulders and arms, promoting relaxation and flexibility. Addressing the psoas muscle benefits your upper back by alleviating stress on the spine, encouraging a balanced posture, and aiding in upper body movement coordination.

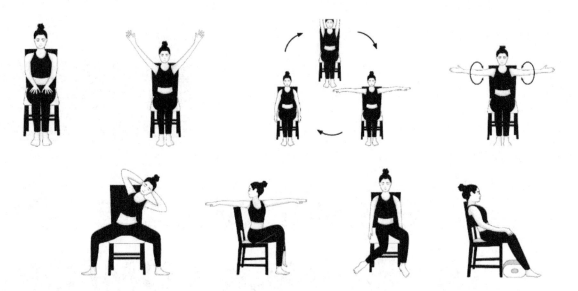

Seated Five-Pointed Star Pose Chair

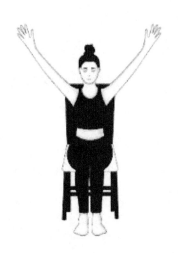

Take a seat in your chair and scoot forward, ensuring your feet rest flat on the floor. Straighten your back and elongate your spine. Tuck in your chin gently and draw your shoulders down while keeping your ears away from them. As you inhale, raise your arms up in a "Y" shape, spreading your fingers wide. As you exhale, slowly lower your arms and loosely clench your fists. Inhale again and lift your arms while spreading your fingers. Repeat this movement pattern five to seven times. Rest and repeat it again. Alternatively, you can lift your arms into a "Y" shape and hold that position for a few breaths before lowering them. Tune into your body and choose the option that brings comfort.

Chair Mountain Pose Sweeping Arms Flow

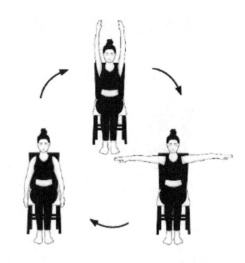

Sit in a mountain pose. Inhale, reaching the arms up, palms facing each other above your head. Exhale and slowly release them down, palms facing down. Inhale, reaching the arms up; exhale with palms facing down. Repeat the sequence for another five times.

Arms to Side Rotations Chair

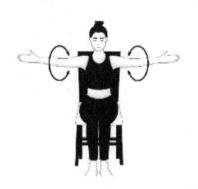

Raise your arms and spread them to the sides parallel to the floor, making a nice T. Breathe in and start making small circles with your wrists in one direction. After a couple of breaths, make a few circles in the opposite direction.

Start making small circles with your arms and slowly increase the motion, making them bigger, and then again, start rotating your arms in the opposite direction and making the circles small until you find stillness.

Goddess Pose Chair Hands behind Head Side Bend

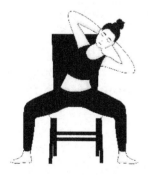

Lengthen your spine, relax your shoulders away from your ears, and settle into the goddess pose—knees and hips comfortably apart. As you breathe in, raise your arms overhead and position them behind your head. Extend away from the floor, maintaining open elbows. Inhale gently, drawing your shoulder blades slightly back. Upon exhaling, engage your core and bend to the right from your torso. You can pause in this position for one or two breaths, or return to the center with your inhale before repeating. Exhale and switch sides. Carry out several rounds on each side for a complete experience.

Seated Revolved Arms Extended Eagle Legs Pose

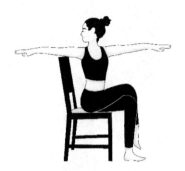

Sit up nice and tall. Pull the shoulders away from the ears and roll the shoulder blades back. Put your right leg over your left leg. On the inhale, lift your heart to the sky. Extend your arms to a T, and on the exhale, twist your torso to the right, the head looking over your right shoulder, arms being straight, at the shoulder level, parallel to the floor. Stay in the pose for three breaths. On the exhale, release. Repeat on the other side.

Seated Windshield Wiper Pose Chair

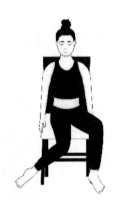

This movement will help you to loosen up your hips and knees. Sit up straight and tall. Keep your legs wide apart. Take a few breaths to the windshield wiper, your knees in and out, moving side to side with your breath at your own pace, releasing the tension. Come back to the center.

Seated Corpse Pose Chair Legs Bolster

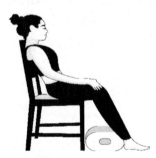

As you conclude your practice, take a moment to sit with your eyes gently closed and your hands resting in your lap. If you need one, use a bolster or make one yourself by rolling up a big towel or a cover. Allow your shoulders to naturally relax, easing away from your ears. During this transition into the rest of your day, take the time to absorb all the beautiful benefits of the poses you've just experienced.

Check in with yourself and notice how you feel. Take a deep breath in through your nose, feeling the air travel down your throat and into your belly. Exhale gently through your mouth. Continue this mindful breathing for a couple of minutes, allowing yourself to fully connect with the present moment.

Before you begin moving into the activities of your day, take a few more minutes to absorb the goodness of your practice. Observe your body with a sense of curiosity and acceptance, free from any judgment or effort to change anything. Be fully present, noticing the sensations that exist in this moment.

ABDOMINALS, FEET AND ANKLES, HIPS, AND LOWER BACK WELLNESS

Welcome to Day 13! Engage in abdominal exercises to strengthen your core, which aids in improving posture and supporting better spinal alignment. Addressing feet and ankles promotes better mobility, supporting overall body movement for effective workouts. Hip stretches create flexibility, which is essential for a balanced exercise routine. Lower back activities alleviate tension and discomfort, ensuring you're ready for active sessions.

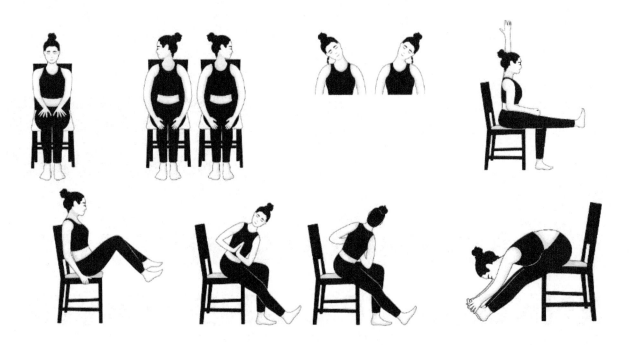

Chair Neck Rolls

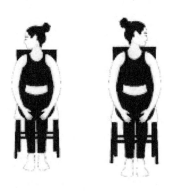

Sit up in a mountain pose to begin your session. Find your center, and take a few relaxed breaths. Inhale, elongate your spine, and feel your sit bones grounding while envisioning the crown of your head reaching upward. Tuck your chin slightly. Inhale, and turn your head to the right, then exhale. Inhale back to center, exhale, and pause before switching sides. Repeat on the other side. Complete this sequence two to four times on each side.

Don't try to lift your shoulder to the ear. You bend your neck as far as your body allows today. Sit tall and straight with your head stacked over your heart and your

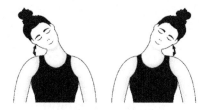

heart over your hips. Feel your feet firmly placed on the ground, hip-distance apart. Leave some space between you and the chair's back.

Inhale, move your ear toward the left shoulder, relax, and exhale. Then, inhale and return to the center. Repeat this movement from neck/ear to shoulders while coordinating breath and movement. Repeat the movement three to five times on each side.

Easy Pose Chair One Leg Opposite Arm Raised

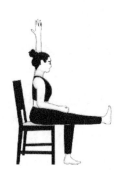

Sit nice and tall, away from the chair back. Use your ocean breath if you can.

Engage your core, and pull the belly button in toward the spine. Inhale and raise the right leg and left arm. Hold for a few breaths. Feel how your leg is activated. Lower the leg, or bend through the knee if it's too challenging. Remember to breathe and coordinate movement with breath. Release to the ground after a couple of breaths. Repeat two to three times for each side.

Boat Pose Variation on Chair

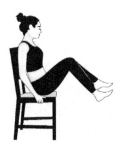

Sit straight and, on the inhale, grab the sides of the chair with your hands, positioning them right behind your buttocks. Curl your four fingers underneath the chair while resting your thumbs near the buttocks. Your weight should be on the outer edges of your palms. As you exhale, lift your feet off the floor while keeping your knees bent. Squeeze your inner thighs to keep your legs together and cross your ankles, aligning them with the chair seat. Inhale and lengthen your spine as you engage your core, and draw your abdomen to bear the weight of your legs. You'll naturally lean back, maintaining an open chest while using your hands on the chair for balance and reducing pressure on the lower back. Stay in this position for two to four breaths, rest, and repeat it again.

Sage Twist I Pose Chair Prayer Hands

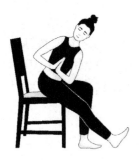

Scoot to the front edge of your chair. Join your palms together at your chest's center in a prayer position. Bend your left leg at a 90-degree angle while extending your right leg, pulling the toes toward you. Maintain a straight spine and an elongated neck. As you exhale, slowly rotate your upper body to the right, inclining forward. Experience the stretch in your calves and back. Hold this pose for three to four breaths. Exhale, and return your upper body to the center.Repeat the same on the opposite side. Repeat twice on each side.

Supported Seated Forward Bend Pose Chair against Wall

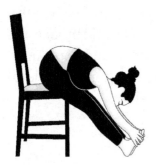

Bring the back of your chair to a wall for support so that the chair doesn't move. Sit toward the edge of the chair. Extend the legs out in front of you. On the inhale, raise your arms, and on the exhale, fold forward till you feel a stretch. There is no need to force your body to go deeper. Hold the position for five full breaths or less. Gently return to a neutral position.

Before completing the routine and continuing with your daily activities, remain seated in a mountain chair position and absorb the practice.

Take a few deep, cleansing breaths. Inhale slowly through your mouth and exhale through your nose. Notice how you feel. Observe your breath. Let each breath flow effortlessly, like the gentle rise and fall of the tide. As you breathe, visualize a sense of calm and tranquility wash over you like a soothing wave. Imagine this peace enveloping your entire being, from the top of your head to the tips of your toes.

Stay in this state of mindfulness for a few moments, savoring the stillness and serenity you've cultivated through your chair yoga practice. When you're ready, gently open your eyes, carry this inner calm, and continue your day with renewed energy and relaxation.

HIP OPENERS, LOWER BACK, AND NECK RELIEF WITH CORE ACTIVATION

Today's sequence focuses on hip openers, lower back comfort, and neck relief. Additionally, I introduced the eagle arms pose, which enhances upper body flexibility and activates your core muscles, contributing to overall strength and stability. With each movement, envision tension melting away and muscles awakening.

You'll find increased mobility, reduced discomfort, and a stronger core through consistent practice. Your commitment to self-care is evident in your dedication to these routines. Keep showing up.

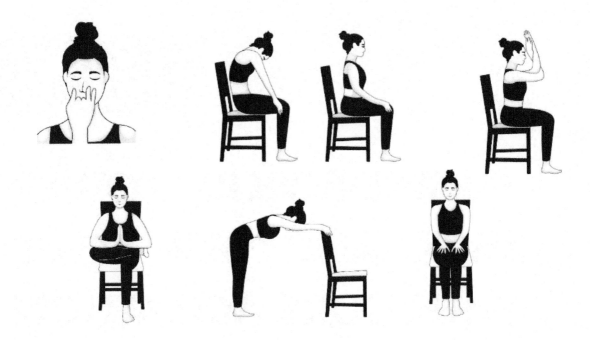

Alternate Nostril Breathing Chair

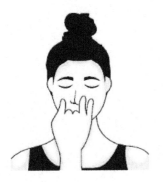

Sit nice and tall in a mountain pose. Rest your left hand on your left thigh or in your lap, or use it to support the elbow of your right arm. Close your right nostril with the thumb of that hand, inhale through the left, and then close it off with your ring finger and pinky. Exhale through the right nostril for a short pause before repeating this cycle three to five times with both nostrils. When finished, return to regular breathing.

Chair Cat-Cow Pose

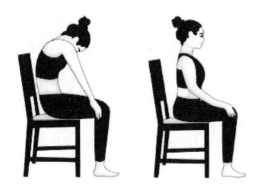

Place your arms on your knees. As you inhale, expand your chest, allowing your head and chin to tilt slightly back. On the exhale, round your spine by curling your chest inward. Ensure your shoulders are relaxed, and be aware of the space between your shoulders and earlobes. Practice coordinating your breath with the movement, moving at a comfortable pace. Repeat five to eight times.

Remember to smile, inhale deeply, and repeat this movement three to five times. Take your time and enjoy the practice.

Eagle Arms

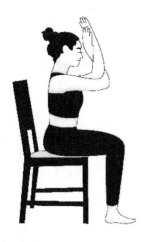

This movement offers a swift means of alleviating shoulder and neck stiffness by stretching the entire back muscles. Find a comfortable seat on a chair, ensuring your back is straight and your feet are securely planted on the floor. Take a few calming breaths in this position. Cross your elbows, placing your right arm over the left.

Link your arms together, and focus on your breath as you hold the position for three breaths. Release and replicate the movement on the other side. Cross your left elbow over the right. Maintain your breath for another three breaths. Then, release and return to the center. Repeat it twice.

Chair Pigeon Pose Variation Forward Bend

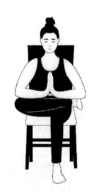

On the inhale, bring the right ankle to rest on the left thigh with your hands, keeping the knee in line with your ankle as much as possible. The left leg is grounded with the flat foot in the chair pigeon pose. Use both hands to adjust the ankle position on the other knee. Breathe and lengthen the spine. Feel the hip flexors contracting and the joints of the hips, knee, and ankle being active. Engage the pelvic floor muscles and remain here for about four to five breaths, consciously pushing the right knee down (but without using the hands). Inhale, and bring the hands in front of your chest, palms facing each other. Keep forearms parallel to the ground. As you exhale, go for a forward bend from the hips to intensify the stretch. Engage the pelvic muscles. Try bringing the chest closer to the thighs. Breathe, and observe how your body feels—moving forward when exhaling. Find the spot until you can't go any farther, and once comfortable, hold for about three to four breaths. If you can, on the exhale, go deeper into the forward bend. If you cannot, then stay where you are. Remember to keep your spine long, your shoulders relaxed, and away from your ears. To release, inhale, lift your head, and come up to straight back, exhale, release the hands, and with the support of hands, release the right leg, and relax. Repeat the same steps on the other side.

Standing Forward Bend Chair

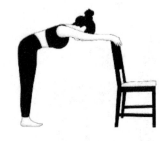

Begin in the mountain pose, elongating your legs and engaging your kneecaps. Extend your arms toward the ceiling with palms facing forward, creating length throughout your entire body. Fold forward from the hips with an exhale, ensuring your legs are extended without locking the knees. Place your palms lightly on a chair about three feet before you. Maintain a parallel alignment between your spine and the floor while gently lifting through your sitting bones. Remember, the chair offers support, but avoid putting all your weight on it. Feel your abdominal muscles engaging to maintain your posture and spinal alignment. Sense the energy radiating through the back of your legs and ensure even pressure on both the inner and outer edges of each foot. Hold this pose for thirty to sixty seconds, gradually aiming for longer durations as you progress. Throughout the practice, maintain steady and even breathing.

HAMSTRINGS, HIPS, KNEES, AND QUADRICEPS CARE

Today, you will work on your hamstrings, hips, knees, and quadriceps. You'll promote flexibility and strength in these interconnected muscle groups through a sequence of purposeful poses.

Engage in gentle movements that address tightness in the hamstrings, promoting better leg flexibility. Hip- and knee-focused exercises encourage mobility and joint health, while quadriceps stretches enhance overall leg functionality.

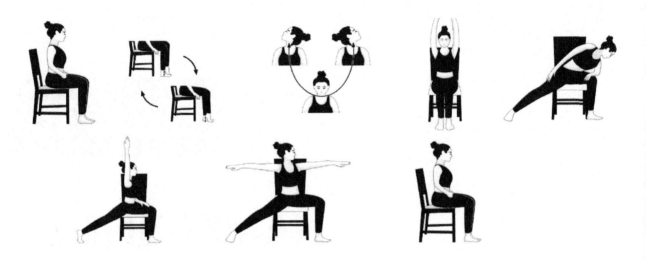

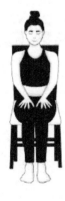

Sit comfortably on the chair and maintain a straight spine. You can lean on your chair backrest—as long as you sit tall with your shoulders lowered. Unbend your arms and stretch out your fingers. This is to imitate a lion's claws. Inhale through the nostrils, then exhale with a loud "ha" from the mouth, extending your tongue as close to the chin as you can. While breathing out, focus on the middle of your forehead or the end of your nose. Fill up with breath, and go back to neutral facial expression. Repeat four to six times.

Chair Mountain Pose Heel Raise

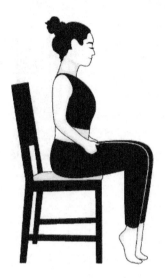

Start with feet flat on the floor. Inhale—lift both heels, pressing the toes into the floor, and lower on the exhale. Repeat five times. Inhale—lift the right heel, pressing the toes into the floor, and lower on the exhale. Repeat five times.Continue by lifting your toes. Inhale—lift your right toes, pressing your heels into the floor and lower on the exhale. Repeat the same with your left foot. Repeat five times for each foot. Lift the toes of both feet at the same time, pressing the heels into the ground. Repeat another five times. Use your deep breath.

Neck U Rotation Close-Up

While the movement may seem simple, the improved range of motion helps with other poses and day-to-day activities. Sit comfortably in the chair with a straight spine and feet on the floor. Let your arms rest at your sides. As you inhale, turn your head to the left, exhale, and tuck your chin toward your chest. Inhaling once more, move your chin toward the right shoulder, and exhale, rolling it back to your chest. Alternate between both sides until you return to a neutral position with the chin parallel to the floor. Stay here for two rounds.

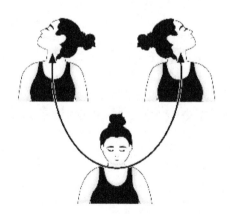

Chair Upward Hand Stretch Pose

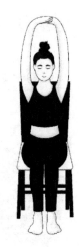

On the inhale, raise your arms above your head and bring the hands in an interlock. On the exhale, try to lower your shoulders. Think about making the spaces between your ears and shoulders. Remain in a stretch position for two to three breaths. Release your arms on the exhale.Repeat it twice.

Extended Side Angle Pose Variation Elbow Chair

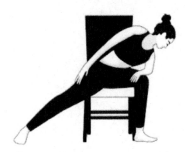

On the inhale, sit sideways, resting the left thigh on the chair while bringing the other leg out. Exhale, stretch the right leg out, and place the right foot on the floor with toes facing forward. Inhale—adjust the left foot, turning it outward, and rest the left hand on the left thigh. Let your right arm rest on the right thigh. Exhale, rotate your chest, and face downward, gazing toward the left side of the ground. Don't let your torso collapse; keep it straight. Stay for three to four breaths. Repeat on the opposite side.

Warrior Pose I Chair Variation

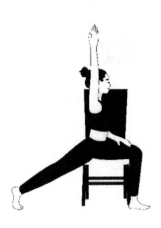

Slide your left leg toward the left side. Let the left leg rest over the edge of the chair while swinging your right leg behind you. Position the sole of your left foot on the floor, roughly parallel to the chair's seat. Straighten your right leg, using your toes for support. If needed, you can slightly bend your right knee. Your upper body is turned toward the left leg, creating a pleasing 90-degree angle with your knee stacked above the ankle. Engage your pelvis, ensuring a straight spine, and lift your heart upward. On an inhale, raise your right arm toward the ceiling while allowing your left forearm to rest on your thigh. Stay for three to four breaths. Repeat on the opposite side.

Warrior Pose II Chair

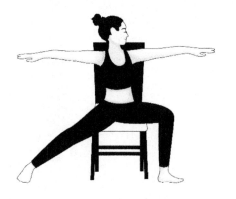

Sit on the edge of the chair. Inhale, and separate the feet. Starting on the left first, open the left leg like a goddess pose, but the left leg only. The knee aligns with the ankle and hip, forming a 90-degree angle. The foot is flat and relaxed, with the toes pointing to the left. Exhale and extend the right leg behind to make it straight in the knee. The right foot is flat here, and the toes point to the front. Make your back straight with your hands resting on the knees. Sit nice and tall. Once the body is comfortable, inhale and extend your arms at shoulder level to a nice T. Ensure the palms are face down and elbows are not bent. Finally, turn your head and gaze at your left fingers. Don't collapse; the torso is straight, and the shoulders are lowered. While here, check the alignment of the legs—the front knee doesn't drop to the side. Stay balanced in the pose. Breathe slowly, deeply, and softly. Stay for three to four breaths.

To release the pose: Turn your head back to the center on the exhale. Lower your hands, and realign your legs to the mountain pose. Stay here for a while. Following the previous steps, counter the stretch on the other side.

To cool down, finish your practice in a mountain pose. Feel the rise and fall of your abdomen with each inhale and exhale. Do five rounds, and feel the ground under your feet. Move your toes and feel each of them. Notice how you feel. Move your fingers and wrist. Observe. Observe your breath. Concentrate on it for a few minutes and, when you're ready, then finish the session.

FEET AND ANKLES RENEWAL — COMPLETING A BALANCED JOURNEY

Welcome to Day 16 of your chair yoga series! Today's routine focuses on renewing your feet and ankles, adding the final touch to a well-balanced journey covering various body parts.

As you engage in gentle stretches and movements for your feet and ankles, you're providing much-needed care to these foundational components of your body. Remember that your feet and ankles support you daily; this practice is your way of expressing gratitude to them.

By addressing these often-neglected areas, you're completing a comprehensive journey that has targeted different muscle groups. Throughout these routines, you've nurtured flexibility, strength, and relaxation in various parts of your body.

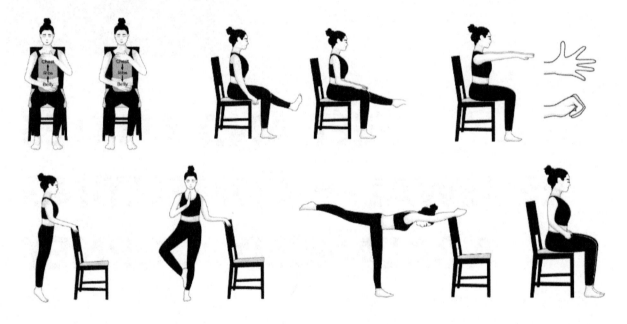

Start in a mountain pose. Feel the rise and fall of your abdomen with each inhale and exhale. Do five rounds, and feel the ground under your feet. Move your toes and feel each of them.

Three Part Breathing

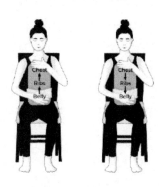

To end the routine, let's practice a breathing exercise. As you begin, you may place your hands on different body parts to feel the air expanding and contracting the area. Begin by inhaling air into your belly, allowing it to expand with each breath in and flatten with each exhale. Take your time to get comfortable with this motion.

Next, take a deep belly breath, and when your belly is expanded, draw in another small breath and focus it into your lower chest. Place your hand on your lower chest to feel it expand. When exhaling, first release the air from your chest, then from your belly, allowing both to deflate completely. Practice this until you feel comfortable with the movement.

Now, breathe into your belly, then into your lower chest, and finally, draw in one last breath to fill the upper chest, expanding it up to the collarbone. Feel your entire chest fully expand. When exhaling, start by releasing the air from your upper chest, then from your lower chest, and finally from your belly. Let each part deflate completely before moving on to the next.

Chair Flexing Foot Pose

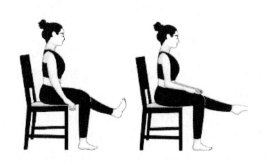

Draw the crown of your head towards the sky and lengthen your spine. Place your hands gently on your knees. Begin by lifting the right leg and pointing the toes away from you. Inhale, lift your toes towards your face, and press the heel away. Exhale and point out the toes. Repeat a couple of rounds before switching the legs. Repeat on the left side. Repeat each leg four to six times. This is a great movement to increase blood flow to the lower extremities of the body, which can aid in reducing leg lymphedema, varicose veins, and other possible discomforts in the calves and feet.

Hand Clenches Chair

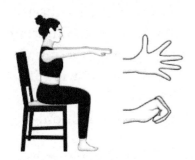

Stretch the arms out and sit up nice and tall. Lift straight arm within shoulder level. Stretch all the fingers out wide open. Close them to make a fist. Breathe deeply. Keep stretching your fingers out and returning them to a fist fifteen times. Take a rest and repeat it.

Heel Raises Chair

Use the chair's support when attempting heel raises if balance poses a challenge. As you inhale, elevate your body, finding equilibrium on your toes, experiencing the sole's gentle stretch. This sensation extends from the hips, emphasizing a seamless connection to the leg stretch as you gradually rise. Maintain this posture for three to six breaths, then release and repeat. If this is too challenging, you can go up and down, as this is also a great way to stretch your feet.

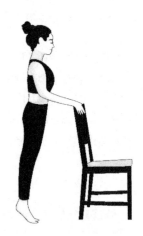

Beginner Tree Pose Chair

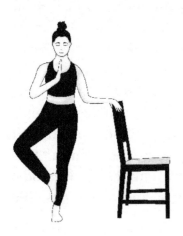

Standing with one hand on the chair for balance, start shifting weight onto the right leg. Ensure your hips stay still. Find a point to gaze at in front of you. Slowly and with concentration, place your other foot against the inside of the standing leg. Bring one or both hands in front of your chest, and the other hand to remain on support if needed. Remain for three to five breaths. Repeat the same on the other side.

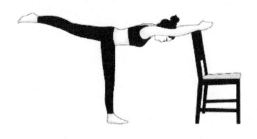

Stand behind the chair, and bring your hands onto the back of it. Come into a half fold. Start to hinge forward from your hips. Softly bend your knees but ground through the left leg. Slowly raise your right leg behind you, no higher than hip height. Keep it straight. Feel your body holding you, and use a chair as a support. Hold for three to six breaths. Repeat the opposite leg—twice on each side.

Complete your session in a chair mountain pose. Observe your breath and how you feel. Think about one thing that you're grateful for. Wigle your toes and feel the support beneath them.

Day 17

HOLISTIC BALANCE
— A FULL BODY JOURNEY

Today's practice embodies a holistic balance, encompassing a variety of muscle groups to ensure a comprehensive workout.

Engage in a sequence of poses that target different areas, including hamstrings, heart openers, hip openers, knees, lower back, pelvis, quadriceps, shoulders, and upper back.

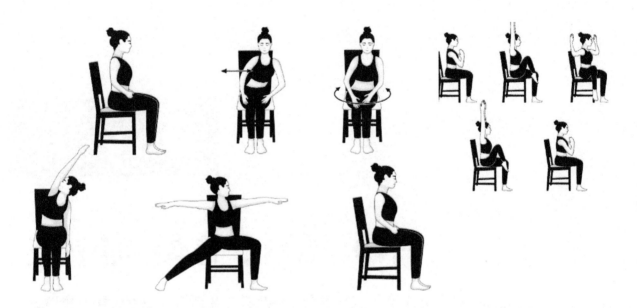

Begin in a mountain pose. You can lean to the back of the chair; however, keep your spine straight, shoulders lowered, and head above your heart. Keep your feet flat on the ground and your spine tall. Softly close your eyes or gaze downward to minimize distractions. Take a deep breath and exhale slowly. Start concentrating on your breath. Notice the sensation. Focus solely on your breath. Scan your body for any tension or discomfort, relaxing those areas with each breath. Engage your hands, moving them mindfully and feeling the sensations in your fingers and palms. Bring your focus back to your breath, following its natural flow in and out of your body. Visualize a warm, radiant light at a chosen point within your body, bringing tranquility to your entire being. Take a few more deep breaths, gradually returning your attention to the present moment. Open your eyes gently, taking a moment to appreciate the calmness and clarity you've cultivated.

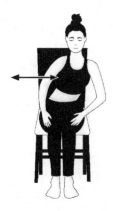

Sit with your feet hip-distance apart or together. Feel your sit bones firmly grounded to the chair. Inhale, rolling your ribs forward. Exhale and round your back, ensuring only the torso moves while your legs stay grounded. Draw circles, adjust the size as needed, and listen to your body. Repeat this movement three to five times at your own breath pace, using deep or ocean breaths. Change direction and repeat the process.

Seated Hip Circles Chair

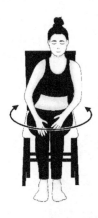

Start by placing your hands on your thighs and straightening your spine. Initiate slow circular motions with your torso, moving from the hips. Gradually increase the size of the circles as you feel comfortable. Begin the circular motion in an anticlockwise direction. Slowly reduce the size of the circles, maintaining control and awareness. Return to the center with your chin slightly tucked, bringing your focus to the rhythm of your breath.

Seated Low Lunge Pose

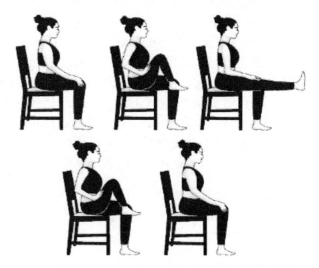

This easy flow will help stretch your feet, ankles, hips, and knees and strengthen your pelvic floor. Sit tall with both feet on the floor and sit bones grounded on the chair. Inhale and bend your right knee toward your chest.

Exhale and extend your leg out. Toes up toward the ceiling. Inhale, and bring it back by bending your right knee toward your chest. Exhale, and place your foot on the floor. Repeat on the other side—a total of five times for each leg. If you need to bend your knee toward your chest, you can grab under the knee and support your move.

Chair Seated Side Stretch Pose

Sit upright. Place the hands on either side of the seat or your lap. Roll your shoulders down the back. Inhale and, pulling in the core, sweep the right arm above the head, creating a lateral bend on the left-hand side. Exhale into the stretch. Allow your chest and head to tilt to the left. Stay in this pose for three breaths. On the inhale, return to the center. Repeat the same with the left side.

You can choose to stay on one side for two to three breaths before switching to the other side, or you may choose to move dynamically between one side and the other on the breath. Do what feels best for your body. Repeat the same with the left side.

During the movement, you may look down at the floor, straight ahead, or up toward the top arm—please choose the option that feels right for your neck. Try to keep your mouth and jaw loose as you move.

Warrior Pose II Chair

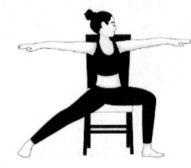

Sit on the edge of the chair. Inhale, and separate the feet. Starting on the left first, open the left leg like a goddess pose, but the left leg only. The knee aligns with the ankle and hip, forming a 90-degree angle. The foot is flat and relaxed, with the toes pointing to the left. Exhale and extend the right leg behind to make it straight in the knee. The right foot is flat here, and the toes point to the front. Make your back straight with your hands resting on the knees. Sit nice and tall. Once the body is comfortable, inhale and extend your arms at shoulder level to a nice T. Ensure the palms are face down and elbows are not bent. Finally, turn your head and gaze at your left fingers. Don't collapse; the torso is straight, and the shoulders are lowered.

While here, check the alignment of the legs—the front knee doesn't drop to the side. Stay balanced in the pose. Breathe slowly, deeply, and softly. Stay for two to three breaths.

To release the pose: Turn your head back to the center on the exhale. Lower your hands, and realign your legs to the mountain pose. Stay here for a while. Following the previous steps, counter the stretch on the other side.

Day 18

NURTURING FEET, ANKLES, HIP OPENERS, AND QUADRICEPS

Today's practice is dedicated to the well-being of your feet, ankles, hip openers, and quadriceps.

Engage in stretches that promote flexibility and comfort in your feet and ankles, which is essential for maintaining a strong foundation. Embrace hip openers that encourage fluidity in your hip joints and alleviate tension, promoting ease of movement. Strengthen and stretch your quadriceps for enhanced leg functionality and overall mobility.

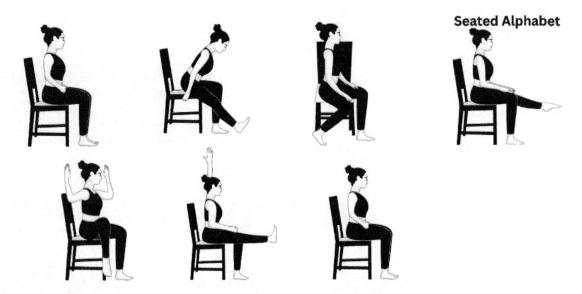

Seated Alphabet

Half Seated Forward Bend Pose Chair

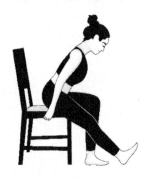

Take a deep, cleansing breath, sitting in a mountain pose. Inhale deeply through your nose, and exhale slowly through your mouth, releasing any tension or stress. Let go of the outside world for now and focus on the present moment as we embark on a journey of relaxation and rejuvenation through gentle movements and breath. Become aware of your surroundings. While seated on the chair, move your thighs forward and extend your right leg, placing the foot out, and resting it on the heels. Point your toes upward, and press the heels firmly to stretch the sole of your foot. Take a moment to feel the sensation of the stretch in the inner sole, and remain in this position, breathing deeply for about six breaths. Focus on extending the quads, hamstrings, and calves, feeling release and relaxation in those areas.

Now, repeat the same sequence with the other leg. Pay attention to the leg with more issues, and try to hold that stretch a bit longer. You can repeat this stretching process multiple times to work on the tendons and tissues around the plantar fascia (ligament) effectively while seated in the half-seated forward bend pose on the chair. After completing both legs, take a moment to relax and settle into your seated position.

After completing both legs, release the stretch and sit back, resting your feet on the floor. Take a moment to relax and settle into your seated position.

Seated Plantar Fascia Stretch Chair

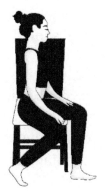

Scoot forward in the chair without going too close to the edge. Keep your right foot planted on the floor, dropping your left knee. Move your left foot underneath you or to the side, toes on the floor, as if standing on tiptoes. Gently push your knee down, stretching your toes and the bottom of your foot. Hold for a few breaths (3–5 breaths).

Slide your left leg straight in front, foot flat on the floor. On an out-breath, lift your foot a couple of inches off the floor. While breathing normally, make ankle circles in each direction for a few breaths. Place your foot back on the floor and slide it next to your right foot. Repeat it on another side.

Ankle Alphabet

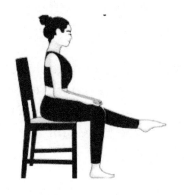

Start from the mountain pose with your feet touching the floor. Straighten your right leg in front of you with your toes pointing forward. Extend your left leg with your toes pointed toward the ceiling. Imagine that you're using your big toe to write alphabet letters. Lift your leg slightly from the floor and draw the letters twice. Repeat with the other leg. Repeat twice, then switch to your other leg. Sit nice and tall in mountain pose. Lift your left foot and place it on the right thigh. Stretch your big toe up and down and to the side with your fingers. Do it ten times and all different directions and then switch the foot.

Seated External Hip Rotation Pose Cactus Arms Chair

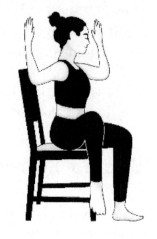

Sit upright, ensuring your shoulders are relaxed and your spine remains straight. Feel a sense of grounding through your hips and feet. Position your arms in a cactus shape, aligning your elbows with your shoulders and stacking your wrists above your elbows. Spread your fingers wide and direct them upward. Inhale, sweep your arms to the sides while keeping your elbows bent, as shown. As you breathe in, engage your core muscles, lengthen your neck, and draw your shoulder blades down your back.

With an inhale, extend your right leg to the right side, and as you exhale, bring it back to the center. Repeat this motion eight to ten times with one leg. If your arms feel fatigued, release the cactus arm position, and take a few breaths in the mountain pose. Then, repeat the sequence on the other side.

Easy Pose Chair One Leg Opposite Arm Raised

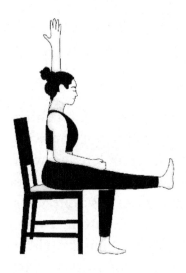

Sit nice and tall, away from the chair back. Use your ocean breath if you can.

Engage your core, and pull the belly button in toward the spine. Inhale and raise the right leg and left arm. Hold for a few breaths. Feel how your leg is activated.

Lower the leg or bend through the knee if it's too challenging. Remember to breathe and coordinate movement with breath. Release to the ground after a couple of breaths. Repeat two to three times for each side.

Day 19

BICEPS TRICEPS, ABS, AND KNEES

Today's sequence is dedicated to nurturing your shoulder arms, upper back, biceps, triceps, abs, and knees.

Engage in stretches that promote flexibility and comfort in your shoulder, arms, and upper back, releasing tension and promoting relaxation. Embrace movements targeting your biceps triceps, contributing to overall strength and stability.

Strengthen your core with poses that engage your abs, fostering stability and balance. Care for your knees with gentle stretches that support joint health and mobility.

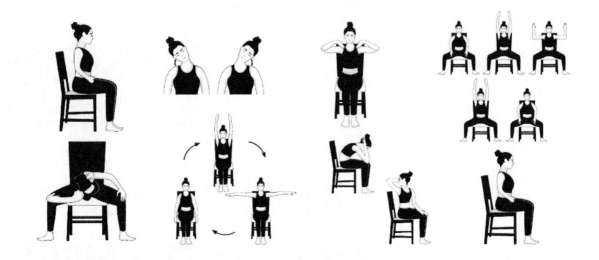

Chair Seated Shoulder Circles

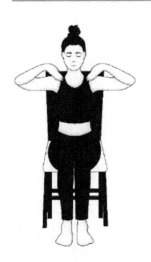

Close your eyes gently if you feel at ease, and take a few deep, cleansing breaths, engaging in abdominal breathing. Inhale deeply through your nose, allowing your abdomen to expand, and exhale slowly through your mouth, releasing any tension or stress. Let go of the outside world for now and focus on the present moment. Sit on the chair facing forward and feet hip-distance apart or together on the floor. Inhale, lift your arms to the side, parallel to the floor. Exhale, and bring fingertips to shoulders. Begin to circle in one direction. Circles can be large or small. Pause and bring attention to your breathing. Circle six to eight times in each direction. Keep your spine straight. Pause, inhale to open your arms, and lower them on the exhale, bringing them to the center.

Chair Neck Rolls

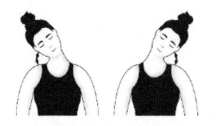

Take a couple of deep breaths.

Inhale and move your ear towards the right shoulder and exhale. Make sure that the neck is long and the shoulders are relaxed and away from the ears. On the inhale, come back to the center, exhale, and pause before switching sides. Repeat on another side, five times on both sides.

Goddess Pose on Chair Arms Flow

Inhale to rotate the hips outward, bringing the feet to 120 degrees, with toes pointing sideways and knees bent. Gently push out the inner thighs as you plant both feet firmly on the floor. Raise your arms overhead—palms facing each other—keeping shoulders away from ears. Exhale while bending elbows so that forearms are perpendicular and palms are facing forward (cactus arms). Hold for thirty seconds before inhaling to extend arms up again with palms together. Lower arms back down at shoulder level in an exhale, and place hands on inner

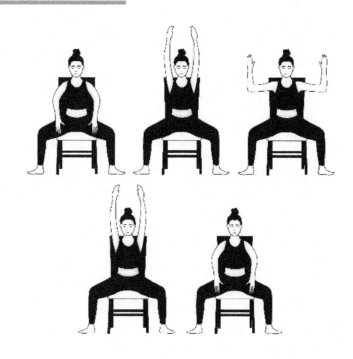

thighs before inhaling again to raise them. Complete four to six repetitions of this flow, coordinating breathing as needed, then release and relax. Once you complete it, remain in the goddess pose for your next pose.

Revolved Goddess Pose

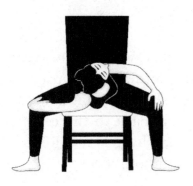

Sit up nice and tall. Pull shoulders away from the ears, shoulder blades going down the back. Check that your knees align with the hips and ankles, forming a 90-degree angle. Place your hand on the thighs. Bring your heels slightly in, and turn the toes slightly out. Roll the shoulders back. Inhale, place your hands on the knees, and slowly bend forward on the exhale, with your back parallel to the ground. Twist to the left first, inhale, and draw the navel into the spine. While exhaling, twist the torso to the left. Take the left shoulder back and the right forward.

Stay here for three to six breaths or as long as comfortable, twisting your neck to fix your gaze over the shoulder. To release, inhale, release the twist and forward bend, and return to the center. Take a few breaths, and as you're ready, exhale and, this time, twist and turn to another side. Bring the right shoulder back and the left forward.

Chair Mountain Pose Sweeping Arms Flow

This will help you to warm up your shoulders. Sit in a mountain pose. Inhale reaching the arms up, palms facing each other above your head. Exhale and slowly release them down, palms facing down. Inhale reaching the arms up; exhale palms face down. Repeat the sequence for another two or three times.

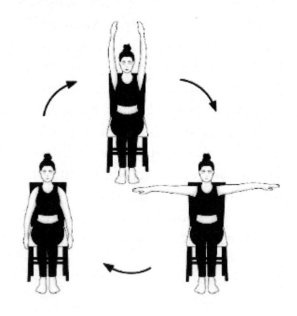

Seated Chair One Hand behind Head Elbow Knee Flow

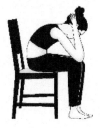
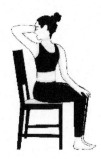

Place your palms with elbows bent at the back of your head. On the exhale, bend forward at the hips, bringing your elbows together, and lean on your knees with your elbows. On the inhale, sit up straight and leave your left arm resting on the thighs. At the same time, bring your right elbow back and look over that elbow. On the exhale, bend forward again, bringing your elbows together.

Inhale—sit up straight once more while bringing your left elbow back and looking over that elbow. Repeat this sequence, coordinating your breath with the movements three to five times.

Day 20

HIP OPENERS, PSOAS MUSCLE, HAMSTRINGS, ABS, AND LOWER BACK HARMONY

Welcome to Day 20 of your chair yoga journey! Today's practice is about cultivating harmony within your hip openers, psoas muscles, hamstrings, abs, and lower back.

Engage in hip-opening stretches that encourage fluidity and release tension in your hips. Pay special attention to your pelvic muscle, which connects your upper and lower body. Stretch your hamstrings for enhanced lower body flexibility.

Strengthen your core with poses that engage your abs, fostering stability and balance. Address your lower back with gentle stretches, promoting comfort and relaxation.

Embrace this opportunity to nurture these essential muscle groups, fostering a harmonious connection between body and mind.

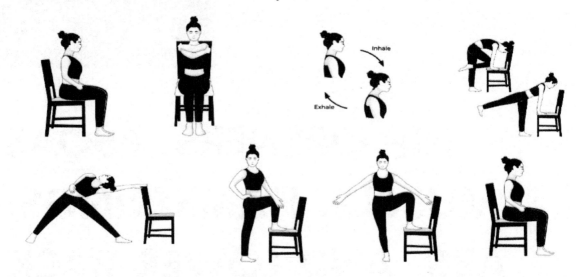

Bear Hug Stretch Pose

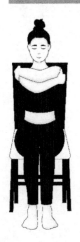

Start by sitting in mountain pose getting ready. Take a few deep breaths.

The hug will help to stretch your upper back and shoulders. On the inhale, hug yourself. Hold on to your shoulders as you open up your upper back while keeping your spine and back straight. Take a couple of deep breaths

Turtle Neck Flow

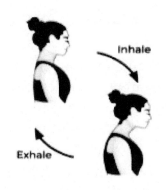

This movement lengthens and strengthens the neck muscles. The neck muscles are connected to the shoulders and back of the thoracic spine. This movement stretches those muscles.

On the inhale, take the chin forward, going beyond the chest and collarbone. Exhale to come back to the center. Repeat it three to six times, making sure the extension is more with each round without moving the shoulders. Don't rush, as the slower you go, the better the sensation of the deeper stretch in tissues of the neck and shoulders.

Standing Table Top Pose With Knee To Nose Flow Chair

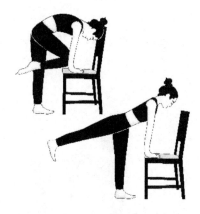

Begin by standing tall and upright, squarely facing the chair seat. Inhale deeply, allowing the breath to steady you. On the exhale, gently place your hands on the chair, creating a supportive connection, envisioning your neck as an extension of your spine. Continue exhaling as you lengthen your spine and direct the extension through your head. Glide your right leg behind you to its fullest extent. As you exhale, draw the right knee toward your nose, curving it inward. Inhale again, send the leg back by extending it, creating length, and then exhale to bring the knee toward your nose again. Repeat this fluid sequence three to six times on one side. Return to your stance in the mountain pose, taking a moment to stand firmly and breathe. Mirror the sequence on the opposite side, maintaining your focus and intention throughout.

Triangle Pose Chair

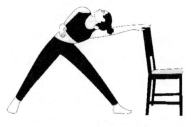

Position yourself about an arm's length behind the chair. Place the chair to your left at arm's distance and gently rest your left hand on it. Inhale as you extend your arm, ensuring your left foot forms a 90-degree angle and the right foot turns slightly inward at 45 degrees. Hold this posture for approximately four to eight breaths before transitioning to the other side.

Standing Twist Chair

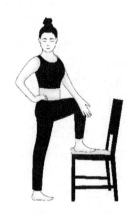

Stand in front of the chair and place your right foot on it, forming a 90-degree angle. Ensure your left standing leg aligns with your hip, toes forward, and knee gently unlocked. Let your left hand rest on the outside of your right knee, and place your right hand on your lower back. On the inhale, elongate your spine upward. On the exhale, engage in a gentle twist toward your bent knee, spiraling your ribs and spine to the right. Hold for three to six breaths. Release, relax, and repeat this sequence on the opposite side.

Tree Pose Chair

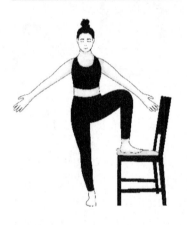

Starting from standing, ground your left foot firmly, and position your right foot onto the chair's seat. Use your right hand on the chair's back for balance if needed. Check your right knee—ensure visibility of your toes/ foot. Adjust for a comfortable 90-degree angle, sparing your knee undue strain and enhancing alignment. Extend your arms like an inverted V, fix your gaze ahead, engage your core, and activate your glutes. Inhale deeply, and if comfortable, gently close your eyes. Exhale fully, bringing your right foot down to meet your left on the floor. Let your hands rest by your sides, palms forward. Mirror this sequence on the left side. Continue for two deep breaths on each side.

Once you finish, sit down in a comfortable seated position in the center of the chair, leaving some space between the back of the chair and your back. Rock back and forth until you locate your sit bones. Keep your feet hip-distance apart and flat on the floor. If you prefer, bring your knees together. Close your eyes or soften your gaze. Bring your attention to your breath, feeling the rise and fall of your chest and the expansion and contraction of your abdomen. Inhale deeply in and out. Inhale while counting to four, hold your breath for four, and exhale, counting to six. If these intervals are too long, do three, three, and four. Continue this rhythmic breathing for two minutes, allowing your body and mind to relax.

Day 21

GENTLE RESTORATION — NECK, BICEPS, HIPS, AND KNEES

Today's practice is a gentle restoration day, focusing on your neck, biceps, hips, and knees. Take this opportunity to give your body a chance to rest and rejuvenate.

Engage in stretches that provide comfort and release tension in your neck, promoting relaxation. Embrace gentle movements that target your biceps, stimulating circulation and flexibility.

Address your hips and knees with mild stretches, encouraging mobility and joint health. Allow yourself to move through each pose with ease, appreciating the refreshing nature of this practice.

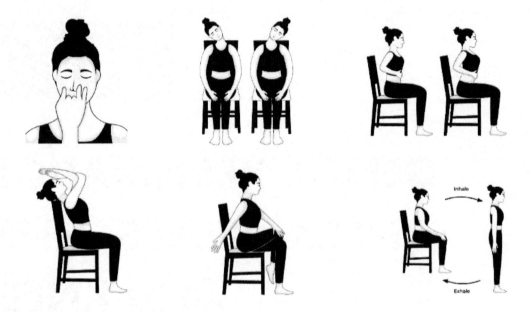

Alternate Nostril Breathing Chair

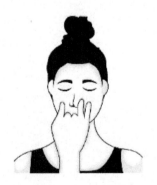

Sit nice and tall in a mountain pose. Rest your left hand on your left thigh or in your lap or use it to support the elbow of your right arm. Close your right nostril with the thumb of that hand, inhale through the left, and then close it off with your ring finger and pinky. Exhale through the right nostril for a short pause before repeating this cycle three to five times with both nostrils. When finished, return to regular breathing.

Chair Neck Rolls

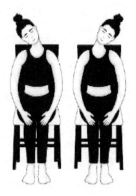

Return to the mountain pose. Find your center, and take a few relaxed breaths. Inhale, elongate your spine, and feel your sit bones grounding while envisioning the crown of your head reaching upward. Tuck your chin slightly. Inhale, and turn your head to the right, then exhale. Inhale back to center, exhale, and pause before switching sides. Repeat on the other side. Complete this sequence two—four times on each side.

Seated Pelvic Tilt Tuck

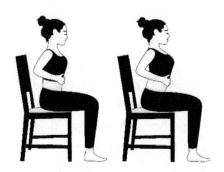

Place feet firmly on the floor in mountain pose, arms resting on your knees, spine erect. Place your hands on top of the pelvis crest to feel the movement. This is a slight movement, just tilting the tailbone back and forth. Inhale as you tilt the pelvis forward, like tipping a bowl full of water ahead. Exhale as you tilt the pelvis backward. Repeat for six to eight cycles.

Seated Backbend with Eagle Arms In Chair

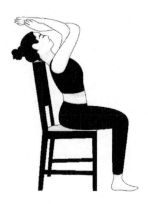

Sit up nice and tall. Commence by sliding your right arm beneath the left, attempting to cross at the elbows. Either clasp your palms or meet the backs of your hands. Elevate your elbows to shoulder height, then guide your forearms outward from your face. Ensure a firm grip as you lift, sensing your shoulders broaden. Maintain steady breathing for a few cycles. You can gently arch your upper back and raise your elbows if comfortable. Switch sides. Remain in the position for 3–4 breaths.

Seated with Eagle Legs Pose Chair Variation

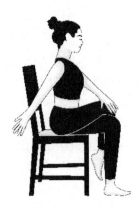

Gently place your right thigh over the left, and if you can, put your foot behind the left calf. Rest your left hand upon your right thigh. Stretch your right arm. Inhale and elongate your spine with each breath in. Exhale as you press the right arm into the chair's back, gently guiding your right thigh with your left hand—within your comfortable range. You don't need to stay in the pose if you cannot at this stage. You can move in and out of it slowly, changing sides. Repeat five times on each side. Or you can remain in the pose for three to five deep breaths and switch sides.

Chair Mountain Pose Standing Flow

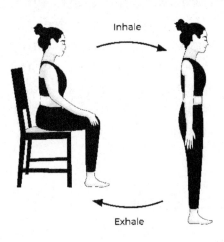

Inhale

Exhale

This is a simple-looking but powerful short sequence to develop strength in the lower body. Engage your thighs and glutes, and on the inhale, stand up, and slowly, on the exhale, sit down. Repeat five times. If you need a challenge, slow down when sitting down—feel your quads and hamstrings in action.

Day 22

HAMSTRINGS, ABS, KNEES, SHOULDERS, AND GLUTEUS STRENGTH

Today's chair yoga routine is dedicated to strengthening your hamstrings, abs, knees, shoulders, and gluteus muscles. Through a series of purposeful poses, you'll engage these muscle groups for enhanced well-being.

Stretch and activate your hamstrings for improved lower body flexibility. Strengthen your core with poses that engage your abs, fostering stability and balance. Care for your knees and shoulders with gentle stretches that support joint health and mobility.

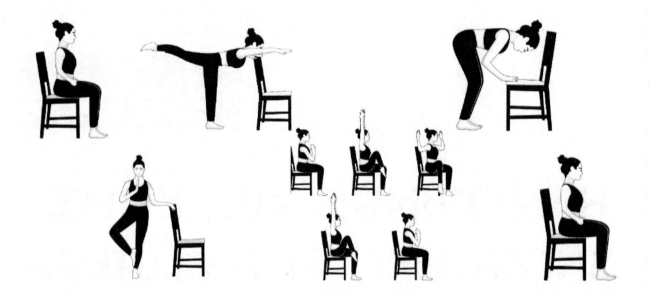

Let's begin in a chair mountain pose. You will perform a so-called "box breathing." It's ratioed breathing that uses a set length of inhalation, breath holds, and exhalations—inhaled and exhaled through the nose. At your own comfortable pace, start to slow and deepen your breathing to a point where you are still breathing easily and without losing your breath. Inhale for four seconds and hold the breath for four seconds. Exhale for four seconds and hold the breath out for seconds. Repeat for three to four times or as much as you need.

Warrior Pose on the Chair

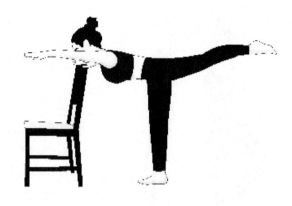

Stand in front of the chair and place both hands on the back. Breathe in, and slowly shift your weight onto your left leg. Extend your right one behind you with your toes touching the floor. Once you find your balance, slowly tip your body forward, raising your right leg and simultaneously raising your left arm. Stay if it's too challenging, then keep both arms on the chair's back. Or raise the arm, but don't fully lift your right leg. Let the tips of the toes touch the floor. Remain in the pose for three to four breaths and switch sides. Focus on your breath.

Standing Push-Ups Pose Chair

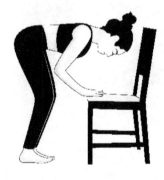

Stand in front of the chair. On the inhale, feel how your spine is lengthening. Bend your knees slightly, and bend at the hip crease on your arms. Arms are under your shoulders, slightly bent through the elbows. Lengthen your spine and neck. Move dynamically in and out as doing push-ups. Bend the elbows, allowing the chest to come closer to the chair. Straighten the arms by pushing into the chair. Repeat five times.

Tree Pose Holding onto Chair

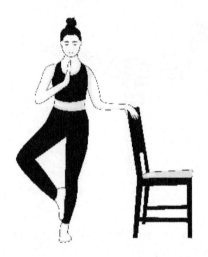

Stand next to the chair. Find a steady point to gaze at in front of you. Move your weight to the leg closest to the support. Square hips to the front, and keep them even with the floor. Place your other foot against the inside of the standing leg—keeping your toes on the floor, calf, or above the knee. Whatever feels right to you. Press the bent knee out gently. Bring one or both hands in front of your chest. Keep one arm on the back of the chair for support if needed. Take three to five breaths and repeat with the opposite side.

Seated Low Lunge Variation Chair Arms Raised Flow

Sit up nice and tall in a mountain position. On the inhale, reach your arms and right knee up together. On the exhale, open your arms to a cactus—arms bend at the elbows at the shoulder level. Simultaneously, bring your right knee to the side. Inhale, and reach both arms back up toward the sky, lifting your knee toward your chest at a center. Exhale, and put your right knee down, returning your arms to the prayer position. Repeat on the other side. Repeat it twice on each side. If you need a challenge—repeat it three times.

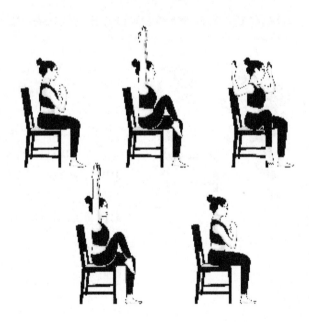

Day 23

COMPREHENSIVE
RENEWAL ROUTINE

The most challenging part is done—you've shown up. Today's practice is a comprehensive renewal encompassing various muscle groups for a refreshing experience.

Engage in stretches to refresh your feet and ankles, promoting comfort and support. Embrace poses that enhance your hamstrings' flexibility and strength. Experience fluidity in your hip joints through hip openers.

Address your knees, lower back, and pelvic muscles with targeted stretches, promoting joint health and alleviating tension. Strengthen your shoulders and arms while addressing upper back discomfort.

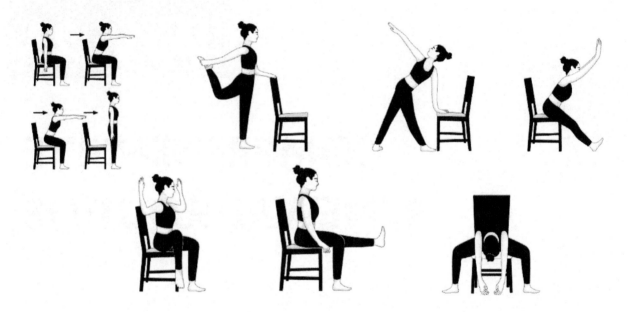

Chair Mountain Pose Stand-Up Flow

Start in a mountain pose. The spine is nice and tall, shoulders rolled back. Take a few breaths and concentrate on coordinating your breath with a movement. Reach your arms forward to help you lift your hips off the chair. Hold this position for a couple of breaths and stand up. Feel the ground under your feet. Sit back down with your arms next to you. Repeat five more times.

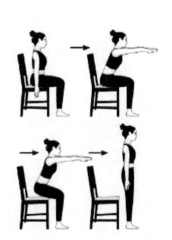

Dancer Pose with Chair

Stand with feet hip-width apart. Engage the core, roll your shoulders back, keep your head neutral, and relax your jaw. Shift weight to the left leg, inhale, and sweep the right arm backward.

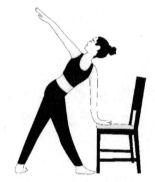

Bend right knee, and grip right foot's instep. Engage the glutes and lift the leg behind, creating traction to open the shoulder. Ensure a moderately bent knee and engage the core for lower back support. Hold, breathe, exhale to stand, then repeat the other side. Hold for three to six breaths.

Revolved Triangle Pose with Chair

Stand, facing the seat of a chair. Step the left foot back. Keep the right foot pointing toward the chair. Turn the left foot out, toes pointing to the left, creating a 90-degree angle between the right and left foot. Take the right hand to the seat of the chair. Rest the left hand on the left hip or reach the left arm to the sky. Hold for three breaths. Bend the right knee and push through the feet with a steady core to release the pose. Repeat it on another side.

Seated Downward Facing Dog Pose Chair

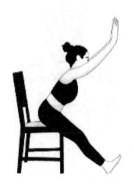

Extend the legs—one at a time. On the inhale, flex the feet toward yourself. Extend the arms up, exhale to lean forward slightly from the hips, hugging the navel in. Think of keeping your back flat. Scoot the sit bones back to help balance. Keep the neck long. Bend your knees slightly if needed. Stay in this position for a few breaths. If required, take a break and repeat it. If this pose is not available, with both legs stretched out, then alternate legs. Pay attention to the leg with more issues, and try to hold that stretch a bit longer. After completing both legs, release the stretch, and sit back, resting your feet on the floor.

Seated External Hip Rotation Pose Cactus Arms Chair

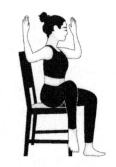

Sit upright, ensuring your shoulders are relaxed and your spine remains straight. Feel a sense of grounding through your hips and feet. Position your arms in a cactus shape, aligning your elbows with your shoulders and stacking your wrists above your elbows. Spread your fingers wide and direct them upward. Inhale, sweep your arms to the sides while keeping your elbows bent, as shown. As you breathe in, engage your core muscles, lengthen your neck, and draw your shoulder blades down your back. With an inhale, extend your right leg to the right side, and as you exhale, bring it back to the center. Repeat this motion eight to ten times with one leg. If your arms feel fatigued, release the cactus arm position, and take a few breaths in the mountain pose. Then, repeat the sequence on the other side.

Easy Pose Chair One Leg Opposite Arm Raised

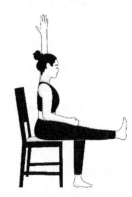

Sit nice and tall, away from the chair back. Use your ocean breath if you can.

Engage your core, and pull the belly button in toward the spine. Inhale and raise the right leg and left arm. Hold for a few breaths. Feel how your leg is activated. Lower the leg or bend through the knee if it's too challenging. Remember to breathe and coordinate movement with breath. Release to the ground after a couple of breaths. Repeat two to three times for each side.

Wide Legged Forward Bend Pose Chair Hands Floor

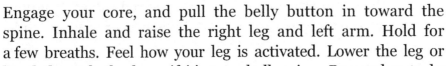

Open legs wide, keeping knees and toes in the same direction. Stack your knees over your ankles. Ground through all four corners of feet. Inhale and raise arms overhead. On the exhale, fold forward. Listen to your body, and go as low as your body lets you. It doesn't matter if it's only a few inches. You can use blocks or a stack of books to bring the floor closer to you. Stay here for three deep breaths. If you're comfortable—remain for longer.

Day 24

COMPREHENSIVE MUSCLE FOCUS

Welcome to Day 24 of your chair yoga journey! Today's practice offers a comprehensive approach, engaging various muscle groups for a well-rounded experience.

This session directs attention to the abs, hamstrings, heart openers, hip openers, knees, lower back, pelvic muscles, quadriceps, and gluteus. Embrace this opportunity to nurture essential muscle groups, fostering a harmonious connection between body and mind.

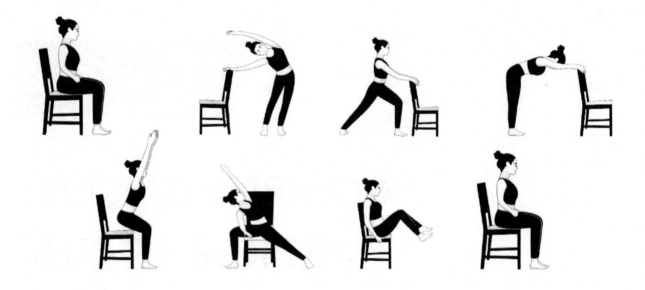

Begin in a mountain pose. You can lean to the back of the chair; however, keep your spine straight and shoulders lowered. Keep your feet flat on the ground and your spine tall. Softly close your eyes or gaze downward to minimize distractions. Take a deep breath and exhale slowly. Start concentrating on your breath. Notice the sensation. Focus solely on your breath. Scan your body for any tension or discomfort, relaxing those areas with each breath. Engage your hands, moving them mindfully and feeling the sensations in your fingers and palms. Bring your focus back to your breath, following its natural flow in and out of your body.

Standing Lateral Side Bend Flexion Chair

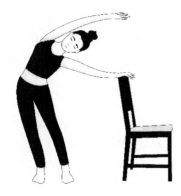

Plant left palm on the back of the chair. Stretch it out, and stand with your back straight and shoulders lowered. On the inhale, raise your right arm overhead.

Exhale and lean toward the left. Look toward your upper arm or look straight in front of you. Feel the lateral stretch. Stay in this position for three to five breaths. If this is too challenging, repeat five times on each side going into and out of the stretch.

Warrior Pose I with Chair in Front

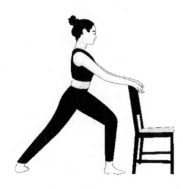

Step your right foot forward, bending the knee and keeping the knee in line with the ankle. Turn your foot at a 45-degree angle, flat on the floor. Square the hips. Keeping the back leg strong and straight, feeling both legs stretched and stable with the chest lifted. Hips are parallel to the shoulders. Remain in the position for three breaths. Repeat the same on the other side. Repeat each side twice.

Standing Forward Bend Chair

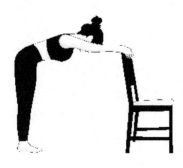

Stand behind the chair. Engage kneecaps by lifting them upward, cultivating height in your stance. Rest both arms on the chair's back. Begin a gentle step back with both legs, finding a comfortable stretch. Raise your arms toward the ceiling, palms forward. Experience a full-body stretch. Take a few deep breaths, and hinge from your waist on the exhale, keeping the legs straight. Distribute your weight between feet. Extend your arms and place palms atop a chair about three feet ahead. Press palms gently, avoiding weight transfer. Sustain length through the back, elongating the spine parallel to the floor.

Chair Pose Hovering Above Chair

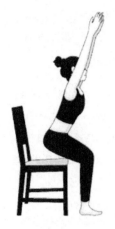

Maintain an upright posture, and lift your arms above your head while exhaling deeply. Inhale and move into a chair pose, gently raising yourself on your feet above the chair. Inhale through your nose, and exhale audibly through your mouth.

Exhale and return to a seated position, arms still extended overhead. Inhale again and resume the chair pose. Repeat this sequence three to six times.

Extended Side Angle Pose Variation Elbow Arm Chair

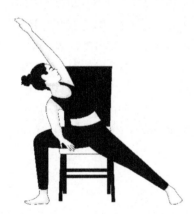

Inhale and turn your right foot outward, placing the right thigh on the chair.

Exhale, extending your left leg to the left side of the chair while lifting your right arm and stretching the side as you gaze upward. Hold the pose for three breaths, inhaling and exhaling deeply. Repeat on the other side.

Boat Pose Variation on Chair

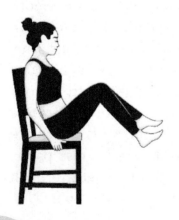

Sit straight and, on the inhale, grab the sides of the chair with your hands, positioning them right behind your buttocks. Curl your four fingers underneath the chair while resting your thumbs near the buttocks. Your weight should be on the outer edges of your palms. As you exhale, lift your feet off the floor while keeping your knees bent. Squeeze your inner thighs to keep your legs together, and cross your ankles, aligning them with the chair seat. Inhale and lengthen your spine as you engage your core, and draw your abdomen to bear the weight of your legs. You'll naturally lean back, maintaining an open chest while using your hands on the chair for balance and reducing pressure on the lower back. Stay in this position for three to four breaths, rest, and repeat it again.

Before you proceed with your day, take a moment to savor the positive energy you've cultivated during this session. Feel the chair beneath you, anchoring you in the present moment. Turn your attention inward with your eyes gently closed or a soft gaze. Tune in to the gentle rhythm of your breath. Release any lingering tension or stress with each breath out, allowing a profound sense of relaxation to wash over you, like a soothing wave caressing the shore. Pause to express gratitude for the dedicated time you've invested in your well-being. Recognize the enduring peace that resides within you, accessible through chair yoga. Now, as you gently open your eyes, carry this newfound serenity with you as you prepare to transition to the next phase with revitalized energy and heightened mindfulness.

Day 25

MUSCLE ACTIVATION

Welcome to Day 25 of your chair yoga journey! If you're reading this, congratulations—your commitment is truly admirable. You've come a long way on this path to wellness and mindfulness.

Embrace poses that activate your knees, encouraging joint health and mobility. Cultivate fluidity in your hip joints through hip openers, enhancing your overall movement. Stretch your hamstrings, promoting flexibility and lower body strength.

Embrace this opportunity to nurture these essential muscle groups, fostering a harmonious connection between body and mind as you work toward your goals.

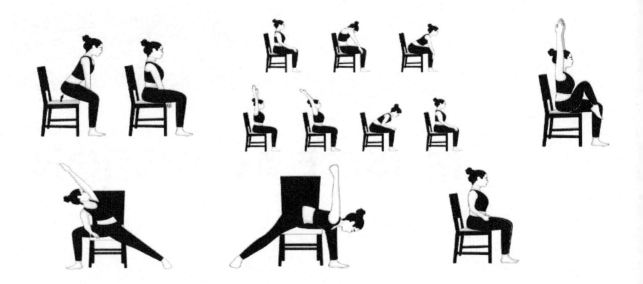

Easy Pose Chair to Chair Pose Flow

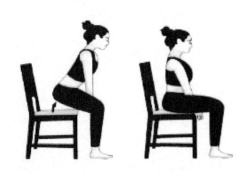

Sit tall, feet flat on the floor, hands on your lap. Take a few breaths to calm your breath, and concentrate on it. Think of the breath and movement coordination. Inhale, lean forward and activate glutes and quads. Lift hips, knees slightly bent. Look ahead, hands on knees. Exhale as you lower yourself to a seated position.Repeat three to five times.

Seated Half Forward Fold Pose Chair Flow

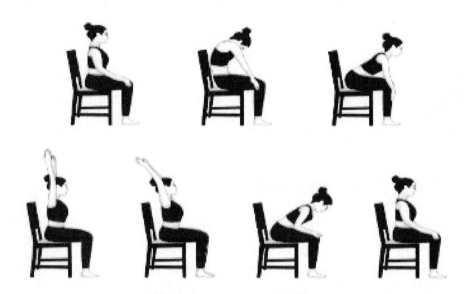

Sit comfortably in a chair, spine tall, and feel grounded on the floor. On the inhale, round your spine, and on the exhale, lean forward. Allow your hands to hold onto your knees, and lean back, arching your back. Inhale, and raise your arms above your head. And if you feel comfortable, slightly lean back. On the exhale, fold over your thighs. Come back to the neutral position. Repeat the sequence two more times. Work with a breath.

Seated Low Lunge Variation Chair Arms Raised

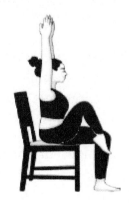

Sit tall with the spine extended. Engage your core. Notice all the muscles that take part in it when you cough. Engage the core with the belly button pulled in. Raise both your arms, and lift one leg and lower. Repeat the opposite side. Repeat three to six times for each leg.

Extended Side Angle Pose Variation Elbow Arm Chair

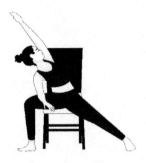

Inhale and turn your right foot outward, placing the right thigh on the chair.

Exhale, extend your left leg to the left side of the chair while lifting your right arm and stretching the side as you gaze upward. Hold the pose for three breaths, inhaling and exhaling deeply. Repeat on the other side.

Humble Warrior Pose Chair

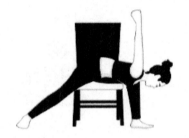

Turn your body to the left with your left leg bent over the chair seat. Place the left leg in an "L" shape. The right leg is stretched out behind you to the right side of the chair, with the foot flat and relaxed and the toes pointing to the front. Extend the spine upward, pulling the belly in and lifting the pelvic floor. Gently interlace your fingers behind your back. Inhale, and expand your chest. And as you exhale, firmly press all four corners of the feet toward the ground. Take another deep breath, pull the arms behind you, and turn the chest and shoulders toward the left side, facing the left foot. As you exhale, bend forward from the hips, gently move toward the left side, keep the chest and shoulders in a twist toward the left, extend the arms behind you upward, and bring the head toward the left foot. Do not droop the neck and head. Think about your neck and head as an extension of your spine.

To release, inhale, look up first, and lift the neck and chest. Inhale, lift the entire torso and come back to the center. With the feet still firmly grounded, release the lock of the hands. Repeat on the opposite side.

Place one hand on your belly and the other on your chest. Feel them moving with each breath in and out, a gentle reminder of the life force within you. Pay close attention to your neck, letting go of any tension accumulated during practice. Are your shoulders relaxed? Allow them to melt away any remaining stress.

Now, take a moment to reflect on how you feel. Notice the subtle changes in your body, the quieting of your mind, and the sense of inner peace that chair yoga has brought you. This is your time to unwind, to let go, and to savor the stillness within.

Day 26

SUN SALUTATION
ON THE CHAIR

Sun salutation variation sitting on a chair combines stretching, strengthening, and breath awareness for various benefits.

It stretches and strengthens muscles, including the spine, arms, and legs. It enhances overall flexibility and lubricates joints.

This sequence promotes conscious breath awareness, improving focus and effectiveness. It supports spinal health and corrects posture issues over time. This routine also calms the nervous system, providing relaxation and stress relief.

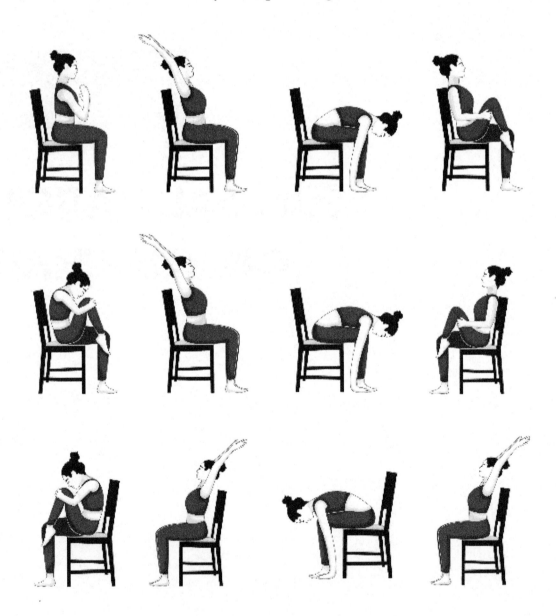

Begin in a mountain pose. You can lean to the back of the chair; however, keep your spine straight and shoulders lowered. Keep your feet flat on the ground and your spine tall. Softly close your eyes or gaze downward to minimize distractions. Take a deep breath and exhale slowly. Start concentrating on your breath. Notice the sensation. Focus solely on your breath. Scan your body for any tension or discomfort, relaxing those areas with each breath. Engage your hands, moving them mindfully and feeling the sensations in your fingers and palms. Bring your focus back to your breath, following its natural flow in and out of your body.

On the inhale, raise your arms. Feel your chest, shoulders, and arms stretching. If you feel comfortable, slightly tilt back. With the exhale from the hips, go forward and fold over your thighs. Stay here for one breath. Slowly come up. With the exhale, lift your right knee and hold it with your hand. Raise the knee toward you and look up. Press the thighs toward you, and bring the head toward the knee with your exhale. Release the leg and rest.

Now, with the inhale, raise the arms. Bend from the hips and fold forward. Stay down for one breath. Slowly come up. Repeat now on the other side. On the exhale, lift your left knee toward you and hold it with your hand; look up. Exhale, press the thighs toward you and bring the head toward the knee. Release the leg and rest. On the inhale, raise your arms, and with the exhale, go down by bending from the hips forward. Slowly come back to the center, and raise your arms up with the inhale. Stay for one more deep breath, and come back to a mountain pose. Repeat the sequence three times.

Day 27

JOYFUL JOINTS

Embark on a journey of gentle movement and tranquility. By focusing on joyfully opening joints, the sequence invites a sense of release and relaxation. The flow benefits various muscle groups, contributing to overall body harmony.

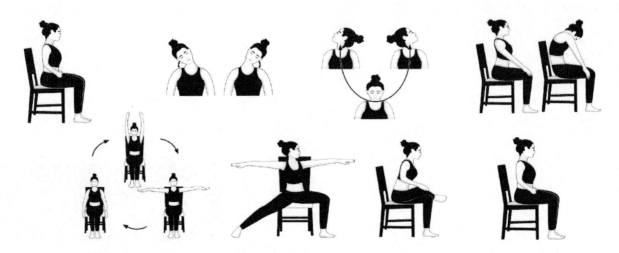

Find a comfortable seated position in the center of the chair, leaving some space between the back of the chair and your back. Rock back and forth until you locate your sit bones. Keep your feet hip-distance apart and flat on the floor. If you prefer, bring your knees together. Take a few deep breaths to center yourself and bring your awareness to the present moment. Begin by gently closing your eyes or softening your gaze. Let go of any distractions and allow your mind to settle. Bring your attention to your breath. Feel the rise and fall of your abdomen with each inhale and exhale. Notice how it feels as it flows in and out of your nose. Follow the breath with your attention, noticing the coolness of the inhale and the warmth of the exhale. Stay for ten breaths, and when ready, move on to the next exercise.

Chair Neck Rolls

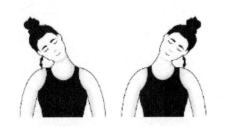

Take a couple of deep breaths. Inhale, move your ear toward the right shoulder, and exhale. Make sure that the neck is long, and the shoulders are relaxed and away from the ears. On the inhale, come back to the center, exhale, and pause before switching sides. Repeat on another side, five times on both sides.

Neck U Rotation Close-Up

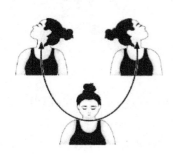

While the movement may seem simple, the improved range of motion helps with other poses and day-to-day activities. Sit comfortably in the chair with a straight spine and feet on the floor. Let your arms rest at your sides. As you inhale, turn your head to the left, exhale, and tuck your chin toward your chest. Inhaling once more, move your chin toward the right shoulder, and exhale, rolling it back to your chest. Alternate between both sides until you return to a neutral position with the chin parallel to the floor. Stay here for two rounds.

Chair Cat-Cow Pose

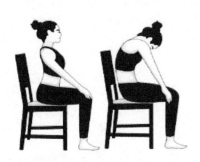

Place your arms on your knees. As you inhale, expand your chest, allowing your head and chin to tilt slightly back. On the exhale, round your spine by curling your chest inward. Ensure your shoulders are relaxed and be aware of the space between your shoulders and earlobes. Practice coordinating your breath with the movement, moving at a comfortable pace. Repeat five to eight times.

Chair Mountain Pose Sweeping Arms Flow

Sit in a mountain pose. Inhale, reaching the arms up, palms facing each other above your head. Exhale and slowly release them down, palms facing down. Inhale, reaching the arms up; exhale with palms facing down. Repeat the sequence for another five times.

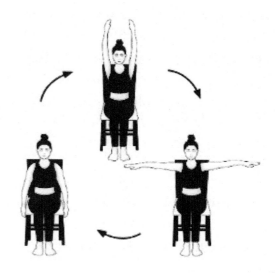

Warrior Pose II Chair

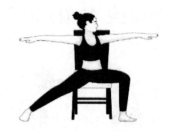

Sit on the edge of the chair. Inhale, and separate the feet. Starting on the left first, open the left leg like a goddess pose, but the left leg only. The knee aligns with the ankle and hip, forming a 90-degree angle. The foot is flat and relaxed, with the toes pointing to the left. Exhale and extend the right leg behind to make it straight in the knee. The right foot is flat here, and the toes point to the front. Make your back straight with your hands resting on the knees. Sit nice and tall. Once the body is comfortable, inhale and extend your arms at shoulder level to a nice T. Ensure the palms are face down and elbows are not bent. Finally, turn your head and gaze at your left fingers. Don't collapse; the torso is straight, and the shoulders are lowered. While here, check the alignment of the legs—the front knee doesn't drop to the side. Stay balanced in the pose. Breathe slowly, deeply, and softly.

To release the pose: Turn your head back to the center on the exhale. Lower your hands, and realign your legs to the mountain pose. Stay here for a while. Following the previous steps, counter the stretch on the other side.

Chair Pigeon Pose

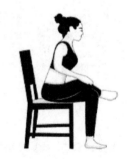

Sit nice and tall, with your back straight. Now, take a deep breath in as you lift your right leg, holding it gently with your hands, and position it over your left thigh, finding a comfortable sitting position. This seated chair pigeon pose serves to enhance the flexibility and fitness of your hip joint and knee through controlled movement. Once settled into the pose, aim to maintain an erect posture, and take three deep breaths or as many as you require to feel at ease. If you encounter difficulty in crossing one leg over the other, alternatively, lift your right leg, cradling it in your arms for a few seconds before gradually releasing it. Repeat this sequence on the opposite side. Repeat it twice on each side.

Pause for a moment and tune into your inner sensations. Observe the gentle shifts in your body, the calming of your thoughts, and the emergence of a serene inner peace courtesy of chair yoga. Embrace this opportunity to relax, release, and savor the tranquility within you. It's your time to unwind and bask in the stillness.

CORE STRENGTHENING AND LOWER BODY CARE

As you reach Day 28, the final day of the yoga series, I hope you've already noticed your incredible progress.

Your flexibility has likely increased, your mobility has improved, and you're generally feeling physically and mentally better. Congratulations on completing this journey to a healthier and happier you!

Today's practice is dedicated to strengthening your core and caring for your lower body. Engage in poses focusing on abs, lower back, knees, pelvis, and quadriceps. With each movement, visualize your core gaining strength and your lower body finding comfort.

Embrace this opportunity to nurture these essential muscle groups, fostering a harmonious connection between body and mind.

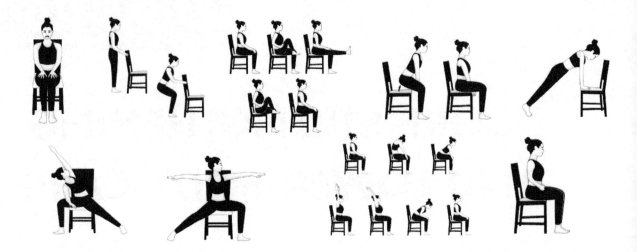

Lions's Breath

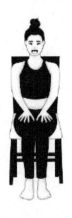

Sit comfortably on the chair and maintain a straight spine. You can lean on your chair backrest—as long as you sit tall with your shoulders lowered. Unbend your arms and stretch out your fingers. This is to imitate a lion's claws. Inhale through the nostrils, then exhale with a loud "ha" from the mouth, extending your tongue as close to the chin as you can. While breathing out, focus on the middle of your forehead or the end of your nose. Fill up with breath, and go back to neutral facial expression. Repeat four to six times.

Let's begin in a mountain pose with your arms pressed against your chest. Take a few deep breaths, and become aware of your surroundings. Breathe in, identify the smell, listen carefully, and identify what you can hear around you. Now, shift your focus to your body. Start from your toes, and slowly scan your way up, paying attention to any sensations, tensions, or areas of tightness that you may feel. Take a few moments to breathe into those areas, and release any tension or discomfort. When ready—move on to the next step.

Mountain Pose Chair to Chair Pose Flow

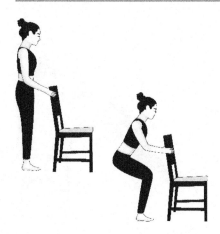

Stand at the back of the chair, holding onto the sides of the chair if help with balance is needed. Inhale, stand tall, grounding down into the soles of the feet, extending the spine upward. Exhale and sit weight back into heels. If you need a bigger challenge—your toes can be lifted to exaggerate the weight in the heels. Lower belly pulled in. The knees should be positioned behind the toes. Keep length in the spine and the back of the neck. Hold for three breaths. Repeat twice.

Seated Low Lunge Pose

This easy flow will help stretch your feet, ankles, hips, and knees and strengthen your pelvic floor. Sit tall with both feet on the floor and sit bones grounded on the chair. Inhale, and bend your right knee toward your chest.

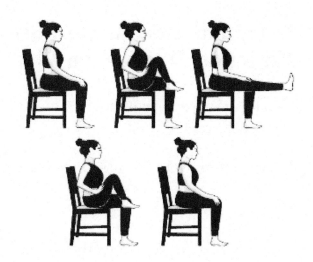

Exhale, and extend your leg out. Toes up toward the ceiling. Inhale, and bring it back by bending your right knee toward your chest. Exhale, and place your foot on the floor. Repeat on the other side—a total of five times for each leg. If you need to bend your knee toward your chest, you can grab under the knee and support your move.

Easy Pose Chair to Chair Pose Flow

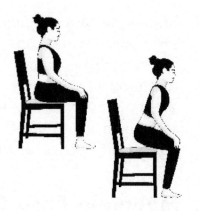

Sit tall, feet flat on the floor, hands on your lap. Inhale and lean forward, activating the glutes and quads. Lift hips, knees slightly bent. Look ahead, hands on knees. Exhale, lower to the seat. Repeat five times.

Plank Pose with Chair

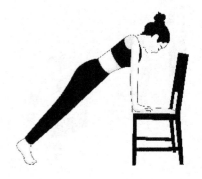

Place your hands on the seat of the chair. Stack shoulders over hands, walk your feet back, hip-distance apart. Depending on your body's abilities, walk your feet as far as you feel comfortable. You can be on your toes or feet flat, core engaged. Observe your shoulders being stacked over your wrists. Keep your spine straight. Long line from shoulders to feet. Hold five long, deep breaths or less.

Extended Side Angle Pose Variation Elbow Arm Chair

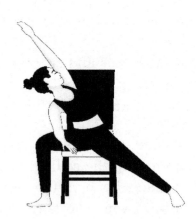

Inhale, turn your right foot outward and place the right thigh on the chair.

Exhale, extend your left leg to the left side of the chair while lifting your right arm and stretching the side as you gaze upward.

Hold the pose for three breaths, inhaling and exhaling deeply. Repeat on the other side.

Warrior Pose II Chair

Sit on the edge of the chair. Inhale, and separate the feet. Starting on the left first, open the left leg like a goddess pose, but the left leg only. The knee aligns with the ankle and hip, forming a 90-degree angle. The foot is flat and relaxed, with the toes pointing to the left. Exhale and extend the right leg behind to make it straight in the knee. The right foot is flat here, and the toes point to the front.

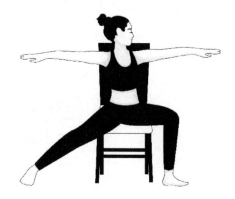

Make your back straight with your hands resting on the knees. Sit nice and tall. Once the body is comfortable, inhale and extend your arms at shoulder level to a nice T.

Ensure the palms are face down and elbows are not bent.

Finally, turn your head and gaze at your left fingers. Don't collapse; the torso is straight, and the shoulders are lowered.

While here, check the alignment of the legs—the front knee doesn't drop to the side. Stay balanced in the pose. Breathe slowly, deeply, and softly.

To release the pose:

- Turn your head back to the center on the exhale.
- Lower your hands and realign your legs to the mountain pose.
- Stay here for a while.
- Following the previous steps, counter the stretch on the other side.

Seated Half Forward Fold Pose Chair Flow

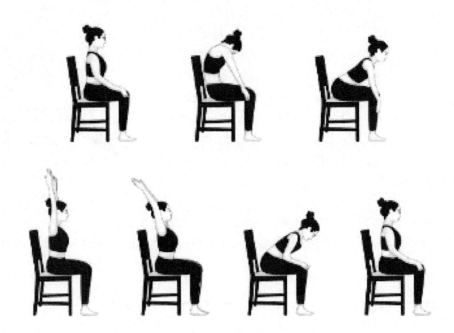

Sit comfortably in a chair, spine tall, and feel grounded on the floor. On the inhale, round your spine, and on the exhale, lean forward. Allow your hands to hold onto your knees, and lean back, arching your back. Inhale, and raise your arms above your head. And if you feel comfortable, slightly lean back. On the exhale, fold over your thighs. Come back to the neutral position. Repeat the sequence. Work with a breath.

Before you move on to other things, savor the good you've done during this session. Feel the support of the chair beneath you, grounding you in the present moment. Close your eyes gently, keep a soft gaze, and focus inward. Be aware of the rhythm of your breath. Notice how gently your chest and abdomen rise and fall with each inhale and exhale. Allow any remaining tension or stress to melt away with every breath out, leaving you in a state of profound relaxation. Imagine a sense of calm washing over you, like a gentle wave lapping at the shore. Take a moment to express gratitude for your dedicated time to yourself and your well-being. Recognize the peace that resides within you, always accessible through the practice of chair yoga. Now, gently open your eyes, carry this newfound sense of serenity, and prepare to transition to the next step with renewed energy and mindfulness.

3 Bonus Sequences

As you have learned, all the routines start with being aware of the present: check if the shoulders are relaxed, keep your spine straight, and guide your attention to your breath. Sit nice and tall in a mountain pose position, feeling the chair supporting your body. Bring your thoughts into the present moment, leaving any distractions or worries behind. Take a few deep, grounding breaths, inhaling positivity and exhaling tension. Once you're ready, proceed with the next exercise.

When you conclude your chair yoga sequence, use one of the breathing techniques you've learned during this 28-day chair yoga journey. You can do alternate nostril breathing, Lion's Breath, or three-part breathing—whichever resonates with you today. These techniques will help you further relax your body and mind. Or you can sit and take a moment to bask in the serenity that your practice has cultivated. Feel your body, scan for any lingering tension, and observe how it may have shifted during your session. Embrace this newfound sense of peace and mindfulness. When you're ready, gently open your eyes, knowing you can carry this tranquility with you as you continue your day.

First: Muscle Activation
Hip Openers, Knees, Pelvic, Quadriceps, Shoulders, and Upper Back

Embrace hip openness for mobility and tension release. Show your knees some gentle care for flexibility. Nourish your pelvic region to enhance core balance. Strengthen and stretch quadriceps for lower body power. Extend flexibility to shoulders and arms, relieving upper body tension. Find upper back relief through mindful stretches.

Each movement enriches your muscles with vitality. This routine harmonizes diverse muscle groups, nurturing both body and mind in perfect unity.

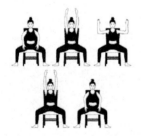
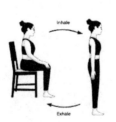
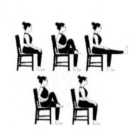

Goddess Pose on Chair Arms Flow

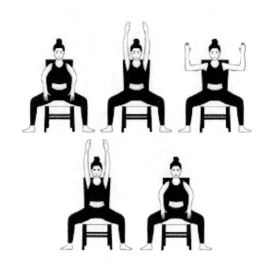

Inhale to rotate the hips outward, bringing the feet to 120 degrees, with toes pointing sideways and knees bent. Gently push out the inner thighs as you plant both feet firmly on the floor. Raise your arms overhead—palms facing each other—keeping shoulders away from ears. Exhale while bending elbows so forearms are perpendicular and palms are facing forward (cactus arms). Hold for thirty seconds before inhaling to extend arms up again with palms together. Lower arms back down at shoulder level in an exhale, and place hands on inner thighs before inhaling again to raise them. Complete four to six repetitions of this flow, coordinating breathing as needed, then release and relax.

Chair Mountain Pose Standing Flow

This is a simple-looking but powerful short sequence to develop strength in the lower body. Engage your thighs and glutes, and on the inhale, stand up and slowly, on the exhale, sit down. Repeat five times. If you need a challenge, slow down when sitting down—feel your quads and hamstrings in action.

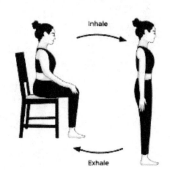

Seated Low Lunge Pose

This easy flow will help stretch your feet, ankles, hips, and knees and strengthen your pelvic floor. Sit tall with both feet on the floor and sit bones grounded on the chair. Inhale, and bend your right knee toward your chest.

Exhale, and extend your leg out. Toes up toward the ceiling. Inhale, and bring it back by bending your right knee toward your chest. Exhale, and place your foot on the floor. Repeat on the other side—a total of five times for each leg. If you need to bend your knee toward your chest, you can grab under the knee and support your move.

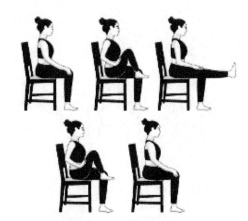

Seated Chair One Hand Behind Head Elbow Knee Flow

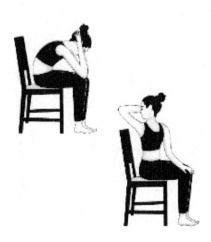

Place your palms with elbows bent at the back of your head. On the exhale, bend forward at the hips, bringing your elbows together, and lean on your knees with your elbows. On the inhale, sit up straight and leave your left arm resting on the thighs. At the same time, bring your right elbow back and look over that elbow. On the exhale, bend forward again, bringing your elbows together.

Inhale—sit up straight once more while bringing your left elbow back and look over that elbow. Repeat this sequence, coordinating your breath with the movements four times.

Second: Balanced Muscle Engagement Abs, Knees, Quadriceps, and Shoulder Arms

Immerse yourself in a chair yoga routine meticulously curated to activate essential muscle groups.

Strengthen your core, cultivating stability and balance. Tenderly nurture knee health with stretches that enhance flexibility. Strengthen and stretch these vital leg muscles for overall lower body well-being. Elevate upper body flexibility and stability, releasing tension.

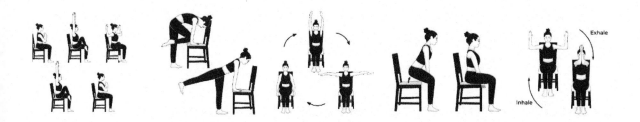

Seated Low Lunge Variation Chair Arms Raised Flow

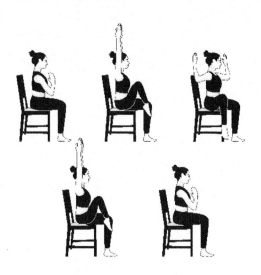

Sit up nice and tall in a mountain position. On the inhale, reach your arms and right knee up together. On the exhale, open your arms to a cactus position—arms bend at the elbows at the shoulder level. Simultaneously, bring your right knee to the side. Inhale, and reach both arms back up toward the sky, lifting your knee toward your chest at a center. Exhale, and put your right knee down, returning your arms to the prayer position. Repeat on the other side. Repeat it twice on each side. If you need a challenge—repeat it three times.

Standing Table Top Pose with Knee to Nose Flow Chair

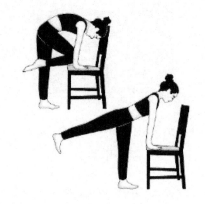

Begin by standing tall and upright, squarely facing the chair seat. Inhale deeply, allowing the breath to steady you. On the exhale, gently place your hands on the chair, creating a supportive connection, envisioning your neck as an extension of your spine. Continue exhaling as you lengthen your spine and direct the extension through your head. Glide your right leg behind you to its fullest extent. As you exhale, draw the right knee toward your nose, curving it inward. Inhale again, send the leg back by extending it, creating length, and then exhale to bring the knee toward your nose again. Repeat this fluid sequence a total of six times on one side. Return to your stance in the mountain pose, taking a moment to stand firmly and breathe. Mirror the sequence on the opposite side, maintaining your focus and intention throughout.

Chair Mountain Pose Sweeping Arms Flow

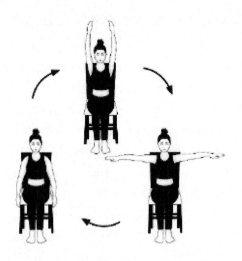

Sit in a mountain pose. Inhale, reaching the arms up, palms facing each other above your head. Exhale and slowly release them down, palms facing down. Inhale, reaching the arms up; exhale with palms facing down. Repeat the sequence for another five times.

Easy Pose Chair to Chair Pose Flow

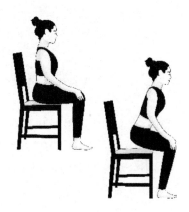

Sit tall, feet flat on the floor, hands on your lap.

Inhale, lean forward and activate glutes and quads. Lift hips, knees slightly bent. Look ahead, hands on knees. Exhale, lower to the seat. Repeat five times.

Seated Cactus Arms Flow Chair

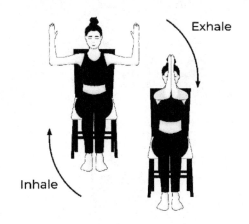

Cactus arms, elbows in line with shoulders, wrists stacked over elbows. Spread the fingers and point them up. Breathe in, and bring your arms to the side with your elbows bent as pictured. Take a deep breath, lift through the chest, and squeeze the shoulder blades together. Listen to your body. As you exhale, bring your elbows, forearms, and hands together. Inhale, open your arms into a cactus position, and squeeze your shoulder blades together. Repeat the flow three to five times. Work on coordinating the flow with the breath.

Third: Revitalizing Foundation Feet and Ankles, Hip Openers

Embark on a chair yoga routine that rejuvenates your body's foundation and promotes fluid movement. Embrace stretches that provide comfort and support to these essential areas. Cultivate fluidity and ease in your hip joints, enhancing overall mobility.

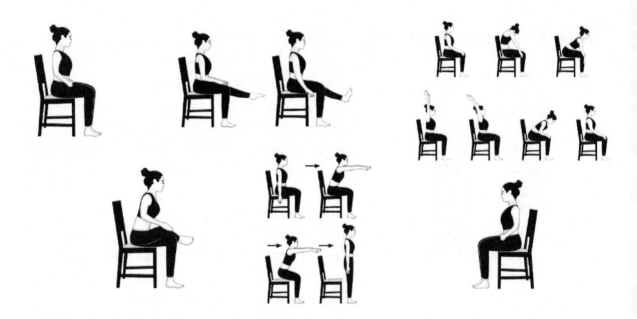

Chair Flexing Foot Pose

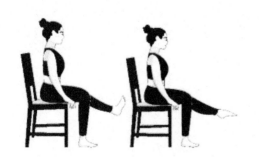

Lift your right leg, and point the toes away from you. As you inhale, lift your toes toward your face and press the heel away. Exhale, and point your toes outward. Repeat this sequence five times before switching to the other leg.

Seated Half Forward Fold Pose Chair Flow

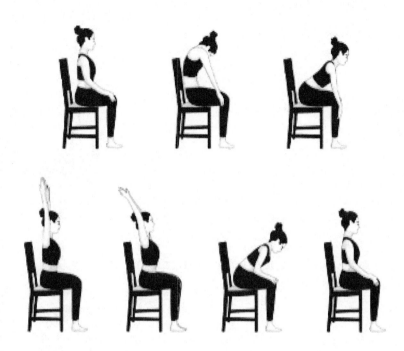

Sit comfortably in a chair, spine tall, and feel grounded on the floor. On the inhale, round your spine, and on the exhale, lean forward. Allow your hands to hold onto your knees, and lean back, arching your back. Inhale, and raise your arms above your head. And if you feel comfortable, slightly lean back. On the exhale, fold over your thighs. Come back to the neutral position. Repeat the sequence. Work with a breath.

Chair Pigeon Pose

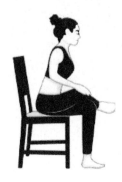

Sit nice and tall, with your back straight. Now, take a deep breath in as you lift your right leg, holding it gently with your hands, and position it over your left thigh, finding a comfortable sitting position. This seated chair pigeon pose serves to enhance the flexibility and fitness of your hip joint and knee through controlled movement. Once settled into the pose, aim to maintain an erect posture, and take three deep breaths or as many as you require to feel at ease. If you encounter difficulty in crossing one leg over the other, alternatively, lift your right leg, cradling it in your arms for a few seconds before gradually releasing it. Repeat this sequence on the opposite side. Repeat it twice on each side.

Chair Mountain Pose Stand-Up Flow

Start in a mountain pose. The spine is nice and tall, shoulders rolled back. Reach your arms forward to help you lift your hips off the chair. Hold this position for a couple of breaths; if not, stand up. Feel the ground under your feet. Sit back down with your arms next to you. Repeat five more times.

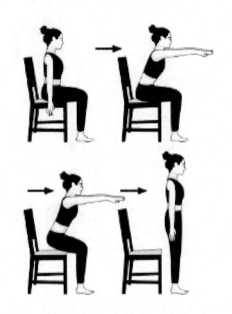

Conclusion

Like anything, yoga takes time and practice to get from good to incredible, and your body is different from everyone else. Use your intuition; stop if it hurts.

Attempting any exercise too extreme (the definition of which changes with age, regardless of fitness) or beyond your fitness level makes injury more likely. This is as true with yoga as any other form of exercise. This is why I actively encourage you—if in doubt —to consult your doctor. If there is any pain—stop it. Don't push if you feel that your body cannot do it.

Chair yoga is more than modified poses. It is about self-awareness. It is about self-acceptance and honesty. When you take those elements out and make it a "sport," with competition, ego, and pushing yourself to the edge as goals, you are likely to hurt yourself.

Each person must find the limit between helping and hurting their own body.

So, whether you follow this program diligently or adapt it to your needs, always remember your "why." Stay consistent, embrace your journey, and respect your body's limits.

As you leave the pages of this guide and continue your chair yoga practice, know that you can transform your life—one gentle pose, one deep breath, and one day at a time. Embrace the benefits of chair yoga, and may it bring you a renewed sense of vitality, strength, and inner peace. Your journey has just begun, and the path ahead has endless possibilities. Chair yoga is your companion on this voyage, guiding you toward a healthier, happier, and more balanced life.

And the last thing before you go: Simply by sharing your honest opinion of this book on Amazon, you'll show other readers that they can benefit too—and exactly where they can find the guidance they need to make sure they do.

Thank you for being so supportive. With your help, I can make sure that the message reaches even more people.

You Could Be Key to Someone Else's Yoga Journey

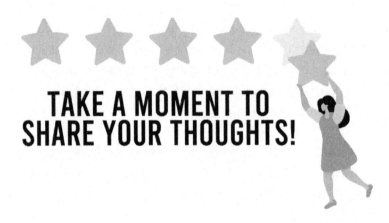

Thank you so much for your support. No matter what might hold us back from standing yoga, we can still access its astounding potential ... And with your help, I can make sure that the message reaches even more people.

Appendix

Day 1: Neck, Shoulder, Arms, and Upper Back Relief

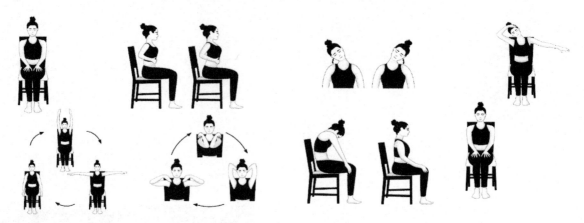

Day 2: Glutes, Lower Back, and Knees Strengthening

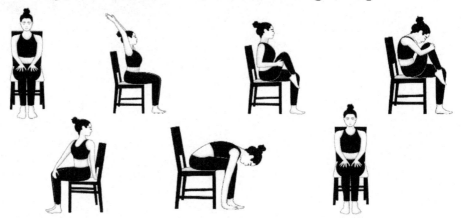

Day 3: Feet, Ankles, Hamstrings, and Quadriceps Care

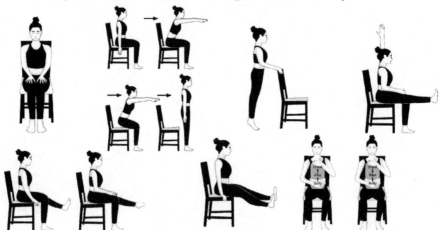

Day 4: Shoulder and Arms Mobility

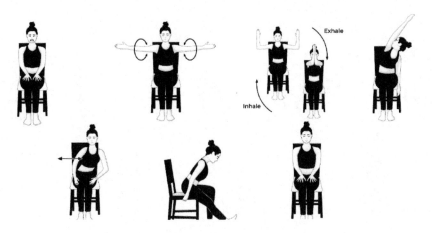

Day 5: Hip Openers, Knees, Upper Back, and Pelvic Release

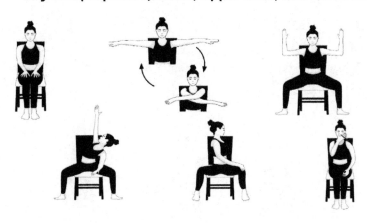

Day 6: Shoulder, Arms, and Wrist Exercises

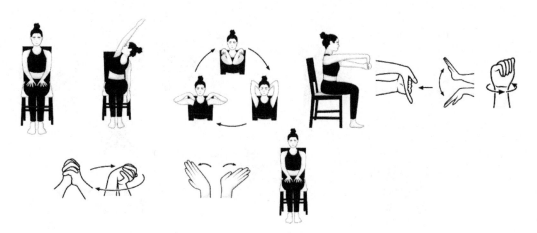

Day 7: Lower Back, Hamstrings, and Neck Relaxation

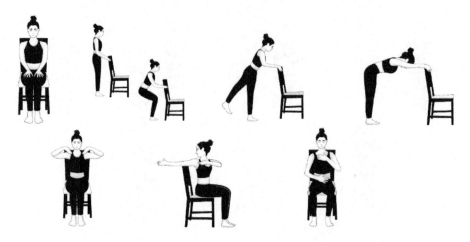

Day 8: Hamstrings, Hip Openers, Quadriceps, and Upper Back Flow

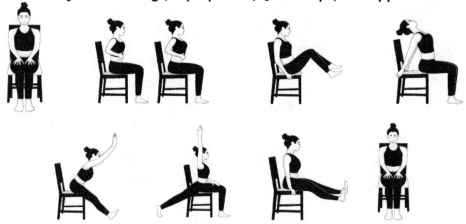

Day 9: Empowering Lower Back, Neck, Shoulders, Arms, and Upper Back

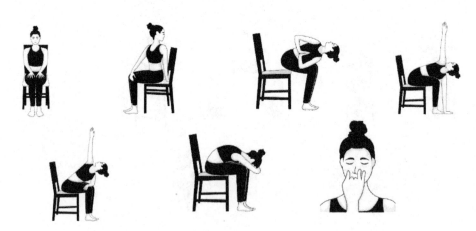

Day 10: Abdominals, Hip Openers, Knees, Quadriceps, and Upper Back Revitalization

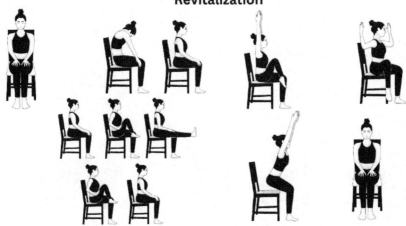

Day 11: Upper Back, Hip, Pelvic, Shoulder, and Arm Harmony

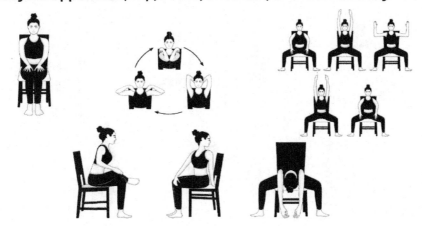

Day 12: Psoas Release for Upper Back Comfort

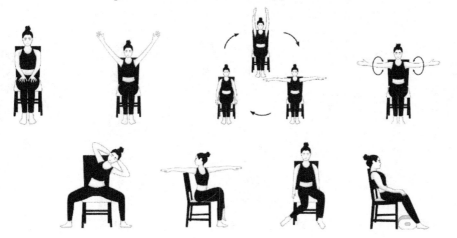

Day 13: Abdominals, Feet and Ankles, Hips, and Lower Back Wellness

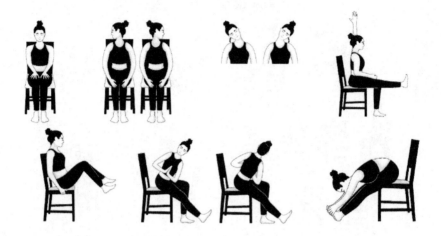

Day 14: Hip Openers, Lower Back, and Neck Relief with Core Activation

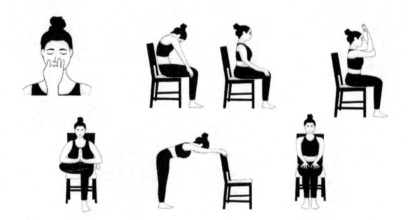

Day 15: Hamstrings, Hips, Knees, and Quadriceps Care

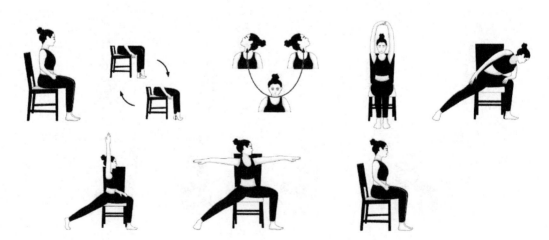

Day 16: Feet and Ankles Renewal – Completing a Balanced Journey

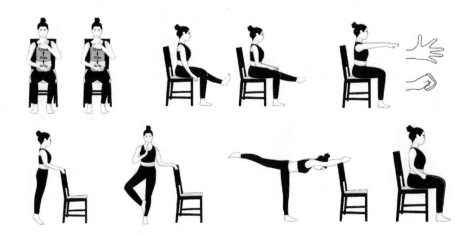

Day 17: Holistic Balance – A Full Body Journey

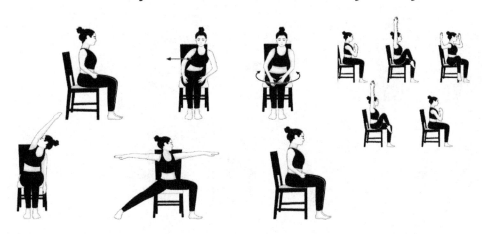

Day 18: Nurturing Feet, Ankles, Hip Openers, and Quadriceps

Seated Alphabet

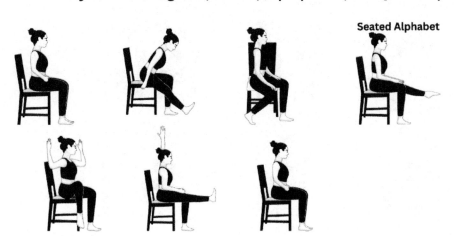

Day 19: Biceps Triceps, Abs, and Knees

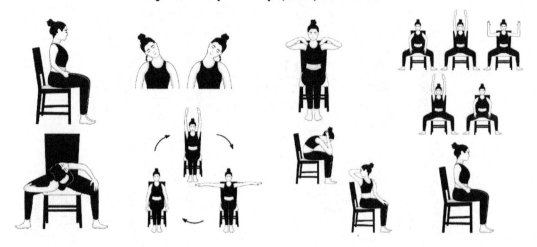

Day 20: Hip Openers, Psoas Muscle, Hamstrings, Abs, and Lower Back Harmony

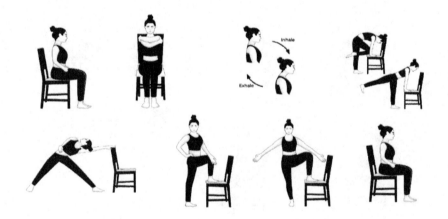

Day 21: Gentle Restoration – Neck, Biceps, Hips, and Knees

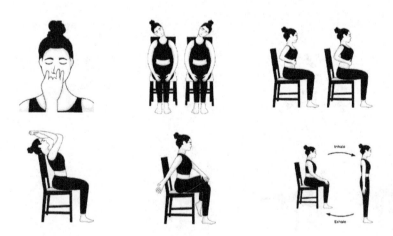

Day 22: Hamstrings, Abs, Knees, Shoulders, and Gluteus Strength

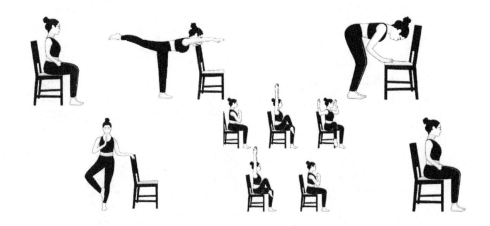

Day 23: Comprehensive Renewal Routine

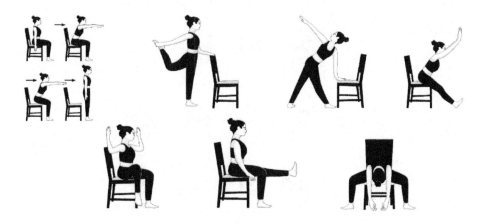

Day 24: Comprehensive Muscle Focus

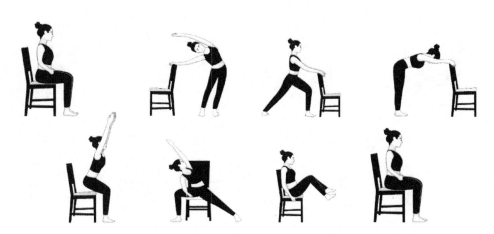

Day 25: Muscle Activation

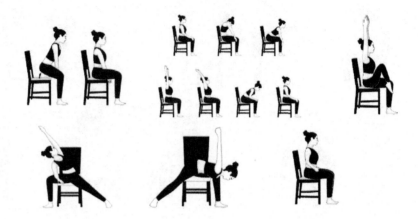

Day 26: - Sun Salutation on the Chair

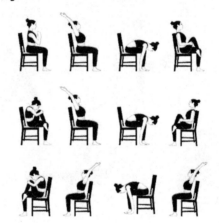

Day 27: Joyful Joints

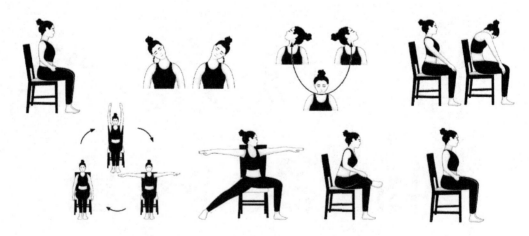

Day 28: Core Strengthening and Lower Body Care

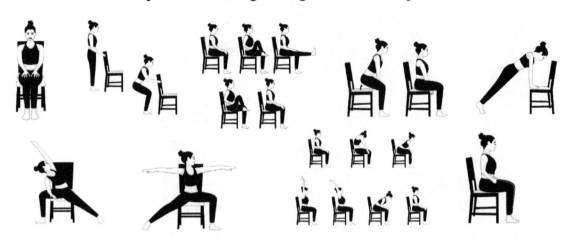

Bonus Sequence

First: Muscle Activation – Hip Openers, Knees, Pelvic, Quadriceps, Shoulders, and Upper Back

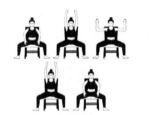 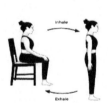 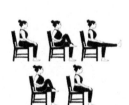 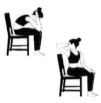

Second: Balanced Muscle Engagement – Abs, Knees, Quadriceps, and Shoulder Arms

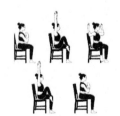 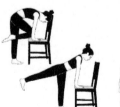 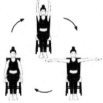 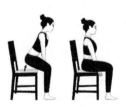 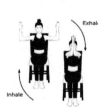

Third: Revitalizing Foundation – Feet and Ankles, Hip Openers

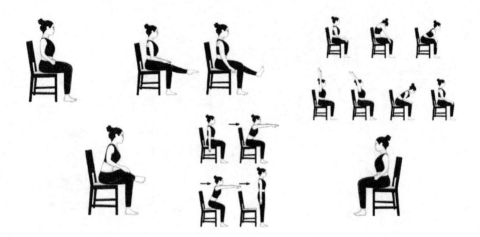

A Gift to Our Readers

I'm thrilled to include a special gift for our readers
15 Guided Meditations.

These 15 guided voice meditations provide a unique opportunity
to enhance your practice. They're designed to be accessible and
convenient for your busy lifestyle.

Unlock the power and experience the countless benefits they offer.

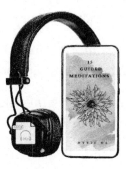

Elevate your practice, enhance your well-being, and embrace the
serenity that awaits you.

Scan QR code or go on

chairyoga.littlegeckopublishing.com

References

Anne, H. (2019, June 17). *7 reasons why warmup and proper breathing is important for yoga*. Simplejoy.co.uk. https://simplejoy.co.uk/2019/06/17/warmup-and-breathing-in-yoga/.

Better Health Channel. (2012). *Ageing — muscles bones and joints*. Vic.gov.au. https://www.bett erhealth.vic.gov.au/health/conditionsandtreatments/ageing-muscles-bones-and-joints.

Bisht, H. (2022, September 28). *Benefits of bhramari pranayama and how to do it*. PharmEasy Blog. https://pharmeasy.in/blog/health-fitness-benefits-of-bhramari-pranayama-and-how-to-do-it/.

Burgin, T. (2012, May 11). *Dirga pranayama*. Yoga Basics. https://www.yogabasics.com/practice/dirga-pranayama/.

Burgin, T. (2021, June 8). *Sama vritti pranayama (box breath or equal breathing)*. Yoga Basics. https://www.yogabasics.com/practice/sama-vritti-pranayama/

Chair yoga for seniors, beginner friendly | Living Maples. (2023, February 12). Living Maples. https://livingmaples.com/mag/chair-yoga-for-seniors/#:~:text=hatha%20yoga.

Cronkleton, E. (2018, August 15). *How to breathe and ways to breathe better*. Healthline. https://www.healthline.com/health/how-to-breathe#stronger-diaphragm.

Excellence in Fitness. (n.d.). *How long does it take for older adults to build muscle?* Excellence in Fitness. Retrieved February 10, 2023, from https://www.excellenceinfitness.com/blog/how-long-does-it-take-for-older-adults-to-build-muscle.

Guillemets, T. (2002). *Yoga quotes (hatha yoga, asanas, etc.)*. Www.quotegarden.com. https://www.quotegarden.com/yoga.html.

Living Maples. (2022, July 2). *Chair yoga for seniors, beginner friendly*. Living Maples. https://livingmaples.com/mag/chair-yoga-for-seniors.

Manning, M. (2021). Exercise the Gentle Way with Chair Yoga for Seniors. *Sixty and Me*. https://sixtyandme.com/benefits-of-chair-yoga-for-seniors/#:~:text=wonderful%20health%20benefits.

MPH, C. A., MD, & MD, N. R. (2021, December 6). *Yoga for weight loss: Benefits beyond burning calories*. Harvard Health. https://www.health.harvard.edu/blog/yoga-for-weight-loss-benefits-beyond-burning-calories-202112062650.

Nunez, K. (2020, May 15). *Pranayama benefits for physical and emotional health*. Healthline. https://www.healthline.com/health/pranayama-benefits#less-stress.

Pal, G. K., Agarwal, A., Shamanna, K., Pal, P., & Nanda, N. (2014). Slow yogic breathing through right and left nostril influences sympathovagal balance, heart rate variability, and cardiovascular risks in young adults. *North American Journal of Medical Sciences*, 6(3), 145. https://www. ncbi.nlm.nih.gov/pmc/articles/PMC3978938/#:~:text=%5B16%2C17%2C18%5D,the%20 representative%20of%20parasympathetic%20activation.

Pat's Chair Yoga. (n.d.). *FAQs*. Pat's Chair Yoga. Retrieved February 10, 2023, from https:// patschairyoga.com/faqs/.

Pizer, A. (2020a, June 3). *Step by step instructions for dirga pranayama three-part breath*. Verywell Fit. https://www.verywellfit.com/three-part-breath-dirga-pranayama-3566762.

Pizer, A. (2020b, June 30). *Easily learn ujjayi breath to deepen your yoga practice*. Verywell Fit. https://www.verywellfit.com/ocean-breath-ujjayi-pranayama-3566763.

Ryt, A. P. (2022). 10 chair yoga poses you can do at home. *Verywell Fit*. https://www. verywellfit.com/chair-yoga-poses-3567189#:~:text=Better%20Posture

Senior Lifestyle. (2020, February 12). *Top 10 chair yoga positions for seniors [infographic]*. Senior Lifestyle. https://www.seniorlifestyle.com/resources/blog/infographic-top-10-chair-yoga-positions-for-seniors.

Stelter, G. (2020, May 29). *7 yoga poses you can do in a chair*. Healthline. https://www.healthline. com/health/fitness-exercise/chair-yoga-for-seniors#Seated-Forward-Bend-(Paschimottanasana).

Stump, M. (2017, June 16). *Yoga and its many benefits*. Lifespan. https://www.lifespan. org/lifespan-living/yoga-and-its-many-benefits.

University of Michigan Health. (n.d.). *Diaphragmatic breathing for GI patients*. Www. uofmhealth.org. https://www.uofmhealth.org/conditions-treatments/digestive-and-liver-health/diaphragmatic-breathing-gi-patients.

WebMD. (2021, October 25). *What to know about alternate-nostril breathing*. WebMD. https://www.webmd.com/balance/what-to-know-about-alternate-nostril-breathing.

Wu, Y., Johnson, B. T., Acabchuk, R. L., Chen, S., Lewis, H. K., Livingston, J., Park, C. L., & Pescatello, L. S. (2019). *Yoga as antihypertensive lifestyle therapy: A systematic review and meta-analysis. Mayo Clinic Proceedings*, 94(3). https://doi.org/10.1016/j. mayocp.2018.09.023.

Yoga for Seniors: benefits, poses, chair yoga | Lifeline Canada. (2023, September 21). Lifeline. https://www.lifeline.ca/en/resources/yoga-for-seniors/#:~:text=back%20pain.

Zerbe, L. (2021, April 21). *Best Chair Yoga for Seniors: A 15 — Minute Routine to Reduce Pain & More* Dr. Axe. https://draxe.com/fitness/chair-yoga-for-seniors/.

Printed in Great Britain
by Amazon